Samadhi and Vastu

The Ultimate Guide to the Different Stages of Samadhi According to the Yoga Sutras of Patanjali and Vastu Shastra for Harmonious Living

Contents

Part 1: Samadhi

Unlocking the Different Stages of Samadhi According to the Yoga Sutras of Patanjali

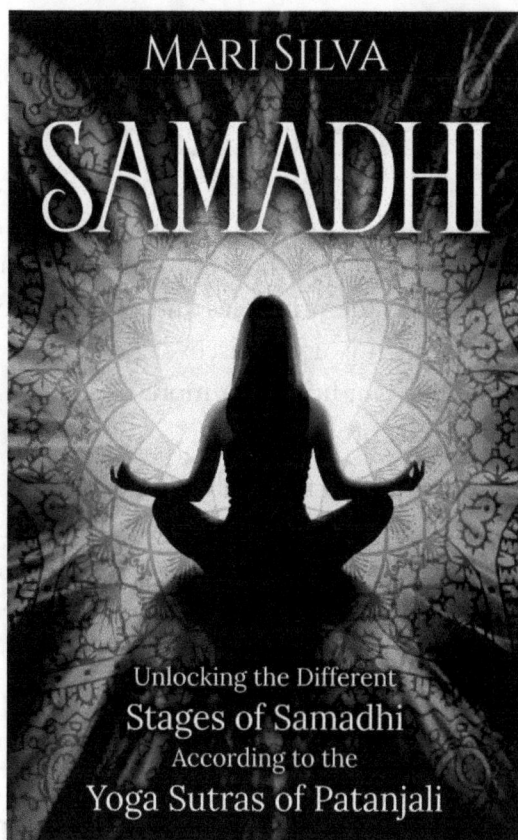

Introduction

Are you interested in practicing yoga but don't know where to start? Or are you a yoga practitioner who wants to know more about this practice and understand the principles and philosophies behind it? If you answered yes, then you will discover how useful it is to study Samadhi, the state that can bring you more happiness, money, and otherworldly things can't provide.

It is the state wherein you have full control of your senses while receiving more than enough power to achieve the divine. When you reach this state of yoga, you will notice your body becoming united with the venerable. It is not easy to achieve and requires dedicated effort, commitment, and practice.

This is where this book, Samadhi: Unlocking the Different Stages of Samadhi According to the Yoga Sutras of Patanjali, can help you. It has up-to-date information about Samadhi to guide you throughout your journey towards trying to attain it. This book is written so even beginners can easily understand it and is comprehensive.

While you can't force yourself to reach the state of Samadhi, the knowledge this book provides will help you make it happen spontaneously, similar to when meditating. By the end of this book, it will be easy for you to experience Samadhi, which will allow you to become more conscious of your mind.

The state of Samadhi is comparable to deep sleep, except you are fully conscious while you are experiencing Samadhi. Your ability to reach this state makes it possible for you to take full advantage of the power of yoga, not only on your mental and emotional health but also for improving your physical fitness.

PART ONE: Introduction

Chapter 1: Introduction to Yoga Sutras

Whether you are a beginner or an experienced yoga practitioner, you know that yoga holds so much more significance than the things you do on the mat. The poses performed and executed on your mat hold more meaning than what others see and believe.

One thing about yoga that makes it significant to the lives of its practitioners is the yoga sutra. Penned by Patanjali, a famous yoga philosopher, around two thousand to three thousand years ago, the yoga sutras consist of a set of texts designed to guide you in reaching a happier and more satisfied and enlightened life.

Practicing yoga while embracing these sutras drives you to be in a state wherein you will live a life full of happiness, intention, and purpose. This set of meaningful texts can provide ancient wisdom applicable even in the modern world, pushing you in the right direction and giving you fresh perspectives on things.

What Should You Know About Yoga Sutras?

Basically, you can view the yoga sutra as a practical and meaningful textbook serving as your guide during your journey towards attaining peace, happiness, and spiritual enlightenment. Note that yoga's real purpose is to unite your body, soul, spirit, and mind.

Based on. yoga principles, humans tend to suffer due to the illusion that their individual consciousness is separate from Brahman or the universal consciousness. Helped by the yoga sutras, you will be guided during your spiritual journey so you can constantly remind yourself of such an important union and forget the illusion of separation.

Composed of 196 truths (texts or aphorisms) – with each tackling a unique steppingstone and bringing you closer to enlightenment through yoga, you will get what you want from the practice. The 196 texts in the yoga sutras are only simple and short verses, but they have full and in-depth meaning. Each text provides practical wisdom.

If you intend to follow spiritual yoga, you can meditate or study these sutras regularly. You can even put the wisdom conveyed by each text into practice by applying and using it in your daily life. This means applying what you have learned from the sutras even when you are no longer meditating or practicing yoga.

But know, just like other yogic texts, digesting and understanding the sutras and putting them into actual practice requires time, effort, and patience. Still, with dedication and commitment, and the willingness to understand the deeper meaning of each text and their individual application to your daily life, you can finally achieve your desired results from yoga.

The best way to have a clear grasp of the yoga sutras is to find or choose the perfect translation. Note that the texts were originally in Sanskrit, so finding the most appropriate translations is necessary for understanding their meaning. The sutras have been translated so often that some knowledge and principles of Patanjali's teachings have been lost.

The yoga sutras are cryptic yet short sentences. You will have a hard time understanding each one, especially if you do not seek an expert's help. To understand the sutras' meaning, go for those translations presented by equally respected and highly renowned sages, like B.K.S. Iyengar, Swami Satchidananda, and Swami Jnaneshyara Bharati.

These men provided the most sensical analysis and translations of the yoga sutras. Just remember these sages have conflicting views, though those different opinions do not arise from them competing. Their individual translations show what their beliefs are regarding the teachings that Patanjali communicates to yoga practitioners.

Who is Patanjali?

It was Patanjali who composed and devised the yoga sutras. While there is only a little information about Patanjali some still presumed that he was an Indian. Most believed that he lived during the 2nd and 4th centuries BC.

Aside from the yoga sutras, Patanjali also gained credits for a couple of other writings, like a commentary on the basic Ayurveda text known as Charaka Samhita and the treatise of Sanskrit grammar called Mahabhasya. Patanjali was also recognized because of three major aspects of knowledge - an incredible psychologist as he imparts yoga knowledge for mind purification, a fantastic doctor for giving people the Ayurveda science for body purification, and grammarian for developing the Mahabhasya designed to purify one's speech.

Sage Patanjali offered the world a nice gift as he brought such a profound and intellectual philosophy into life. Patanjali presented this gift in the form of yoga sutras and in such a way that even the average seeker of spirituality can easily use and follow. So, it is one of those roadmaps that anyone interested in yoga can follow towards reaching enlightenment.

Fortunately, yoga sutras are translated and commented on by many people, making it connect to anyone who seeks happiness and enlightenment from the practice. One of the most famous translations/commentaries of the yoga sutras is that provided by Vyasa.

Vyasa provided the most authoritative commentary, though it is also the hardest to understand, as obscure terminologies accompany it. Despite the somewhat difficult ways of decoding each sutra's meaning, its relevance to the modern yogi is still undeniable. It is still relevant up to today, even when its global release happened more than a thousand years already.

With Patanjali's yoga sutras, you will receive a few important words of wisdom, inspiration, and direction. All these are useful in determining how you can enjoy a more fulfilling and meaningful life.

Chapters of Yoga Sutras

One thing to know about yoga sutras is that they come in four chapters. Sutras means threads, specifically the succinct and elegant threads of knowledge that let you get deeper into yoga's core and essential meaning.

However, there are still a few who continue to debate whether yogis can gain similar benefits from the sutras translated into English than when trying to read them in their original Sanskrit forms. A few controversies as to the number of chapters came out as others say it should be only three since the remaining ones are already redundant.

Despite that, it helps to understand its four originally known chapters, namely:

Samadhi Pada

The focus of this first chapter of the yoga sutras, the Samadhi Pada, is enlightenment. It focuses more on meditation and concentration. Containing around 51 sutras, it tackles the exact process of becoming one. It was named Samadhi Pada because yoga serves as Samadhi's culmination. Patanjali started with the sutras here to enlighten the inner soul of the seeker or Sadhaka.

The sutras in this chapter talk about yoga definitions, the obstacles you might encounter when trying to achieve its benefits, the main purposes of practicing yoga, and how important it is to practice it constantly. The yoga sutras in Samadhi Pada also tackle vairagya, which is all about finding ways to detach yourself from material experiences.

To show you about the sutras in this specific chapter, here are its contents:

 • Yoga sutras 1.1 to 1.4 – focus on defining yoga as far as purifying the mind is concerned.

 • Yoga sutras 1.5 to 1.11 – tackle mental fluctuations diminished or eliminated by yoga. These mental fluctuations include Pranama or right cognition, Viparyaya or misconception, Vikalpa or imagination, Nidra or sleep, and smriti or memory.

 • Yoga sutras 1.12 to 1.16 – detailed explanations on different ways to get into the yoga state, including finding the right balance in serenity and persistence.

• Yoga sutras 1.17 to 1.18 – focus on defining samskara and samadhi – both of which are karma results on different levels.

• Yoga sutras 1.19 to 1.22 – talk about the different types of seekers and the roles played by your memory, will, and devotion during your yoga practice.

• Yoga sutras 1.23 to 1.29 – Here, you will discover the nature of God (Ishvara) and sacred sound (OM) as God's symbol and their significance on your journey when practicing yoga.

• Yoga sutras 1.30 to 1.32 – provide information about the obstacles or challenges you may encounter as a seeker during your yoga journey.

• Yoga sutras 1.33 to 1.39 – different tackle techniques for overcoming such obstacles or challenges.

• Yoga sutras 1.40 to 1.51 – support your journey towards stabilizing yourself from the obstacles, leading to yoga's best experience through various Samadhi.

Sadhana Pada

The next chapter of the yoga sutras is the Sadhana Pada, which is all about the actual practice of the famous yoga. It has 55 sutras, with most providing guidelines and instructions you should follow and adhere to when practicing yoga. It describes the yoga of action called Kriya yoga and the 8-limbed yoga (Ashtanga yoga).

You can see this chapter presenting various techniques and methods designed to remove obstacles gradually along the way. It also tackles major theoretical considerations regarding the yogic practice. In the last part, a few steps or paths to achieving Raja yoga are presented.

To give you an overview of what you can expect from Sadhana Pada, here are some things covered in this chapter:

- Yoga sutras 2.1 to 2.2 – introduce yogis to the Kriya yoga

- Yoga sutras 2.3 to 2.9 – provide information about psychological afflictions or Kleshas

- Yoga sutras 2.10 to 2.11 – offer ways to get rid of any spiritual burden you might be dealing with

- Yoga sutras 2.12 to 2.16 – introduce you to the major causes of Klesha and their individual origins, and their relationship to karma or your deeds and actions

- Yoga sutras 2.17 to 2.26 – let you understand how to treat the major cause of your suffering when practicing yoga, specifically the Klesha

- Yoga sutras 2.27 to 2.29 – introduce you to ashtanga yoga, which covers 8 limbs of yoga

- Yoga sutras 2.30 to 2.45 – explain everything about Niyama and Yama

- Yoga sutras 2.46 to 2.48 – describe Asana

- Yoga sutras 2.49 to 2.52 – summarize the Pranayama concept

- Yoga sutras 2.53 to 2.55 – in-depth explanation of Dharana

Vibhuti Pada

Vibhuti Pada refers to the third chapter of the yoga sutras - with around 56 included here. This chapter is all about power, manifestation, and anticipated results, especially once you reach the desired union. While the second chapter talked about the eight limbs, it focuses more on the six, leaving the last two – the Samadhi and Dhyana – tackled in the third chapter.

Aside from the last two limbs discussed in this chapter, it also emphasizes how effective yoga is in empowering the mind. It makes yogis more knowledgeable about yogic manifestations and powers. It pushes you into the deeper progression of the practice while focusing on the mind's power to manifest.

The following are the sutras stated in Vibhuti Pada:

- Yoga sutras 3.1 to 3.3 – tackle the remaining two to three limbs of yoga

- Yoga sutras 3.4 to 3.9 – define *Samyama* or the art of holding together

- Yoga sutras 3.10 to 3.16 – talk about *Parinama* or transformation and its different types

- Yoga sutras 3.17 to 3.49 – highlight the powers provided by yoga (*Siddhis*)

- Yoga sutras 3.50 to 3.56 – focus on liberation or *Kaivalya*

Kaivalya Pada

This last chapter, the Kaivalya Pada, contains 34 sutras focusing on freedom or liberation, the result that all yoga practitioners are aiming for. It was named Kaivalya, the Sanskrit equivalent of the word detachment or isolation.

It highlights the need to liberate or isolate the soul, detaching it from the physical world's traps, so the main goal of this chapter is to let you achieve absolute, unconditional, and complete freedom or liberation from anything worldly.

The yoga sutras here serve as tools to develop your inner experience while keeping your spirit elevated. It lets you focus more on practicing yoga so that you will achieve wisdom and cultivate the skill of letting inner light guide you through the current moment.

- Yoga sutras 4.1 to 4.3 – cover different ways to reach accomplishment or fulfillment

- Yoga sutras 4.4 to 4.6 – discuss the ability and power of *Chitta*

- Yoga sutras 4.7 to 4.8 – tackle actions and deeds or actions (*karma*)

- Yoga sutras 4.9 to 4.11 – cover explanations on what desires are and their possible consequences

- Yoga sutras 4.12 to 4.14 – highlight the *Tri-Gunas*

- Yoga sutras 4.15 to 4.28 – provide a method to get rid of any challenge or obstacle while trying to reach liberation

- Yoga sutras 4.29 to 4.33 – explain the many changes you will most likely encounter once you reach the phase of liberation

- Yoga sutras 4.34 – tackle the feelings associated with achieving complete liberation (*Kaivalyam)*

Overall, Patanjali's yoga sutras, as well as his story, encompass the development of discipline and mental fortitude – both of which are necessary for your journey towards achieving your desired results. Though these sutras do not cover all the other issues linked to the yoga systems, you can still consider them as classics.

These famous and classic sutras even serve as constant sources of inspiration for all yogis, leading the somewhat never-ending interpretations of their Sanskrit texts. By learning the in-depth meaning of each sutra, attaining your desired genuine happiness and inner peace is possible.

Chapter 2: Ashtanga Yoga: The Pre-Requisites for Samadhi

Ashtanga yoga is a prominently talked about concept in Patanjali's yoga sutras. Encompassing the eight limbs of yoga, Ashtanga is how Patanjali classifies classical yoga. You can see these limbs set out in the sutras, still popular up to the present.

You must commit to mastering these eight limbs or practices in Ashtanga yoga to transcend suffering and identify your real nature. Practicing all eight limbs is necessary for reaching the actual goal of yoga. Remember these limbs follow a sequence starting from the outer (exterior) to the inner (interior).

It is an eightfold path composed of prescriptions for living a purposeful and morally disciplined life. It is also where the yoga postures (asanas) need to form only a single limb.

The Actual Beginning of Ashtanga Yoga

Ashtanga yoga started from the yoga sutras of Patanjali but was further developed into a structure loved and known by many today by two yoga teachers from India named Pattabhi Jois and Krishnamacharya. Famous for holding the title as the grandfather of modern yoga, Krishnamacharya was Pattabhi Jois' teacher. He taught him a sequence of postures or asanas adapted to fit a specific person while still broadly following a similar pattern.

Pattabhi, along with the other students taught by Krishnamacharya, practiced their individual yoga sequences daily following their unique pace. Each session was under the guidance and supervision of their teacher. Krishnamacharya slowly introduced his students to postures that challenge them even more. He introduced new postures to them every time they showed improvement in their endurance, flexibility, and strength.

He also changed every student's individual sequence, thereby challenging them even more. He implemented the traditional means of learning yoga. It did not involve attending a class with a group that follows a similar sequence. Instead, he used a more personalized and customized approach. With the teacher's supervision, guide, and support, students moved and executed poses at their own pace.

Also called the Mysore-style ashtanga yoga, this traditional teaching approach popular in the past often follows a one-on-one setting, allowing the teacher to prescribe a yoga sequence depending on the student's unique needs. After learning from Krishnamacharya, Pattabhi Jois continued applying this teaching approach to a new batch of students.

He gave names to the yoga sequences – the first of which is called the *primary series*. The intermediate series, and the more advanced sequences, namely Advanced A and Advanced B, among many others, followed the primary.

Jois slowly introduced his students to the Ashtanga Yoga's primary series. He committed to tracking a student's progress for ease in identifying readiness to move on to the intermediate and advanced series. This specific teaching and learning setup for

Ashtanga is suitable for the ultimate purpose of the practice, which is to purify the mind and body in accordance with your own pace.

It lets you move comfortably and powerfully while eliminating any extra on your physical and mental health that might interfere with the practice. With that, you can easily follow the 8-fold path or the 8 limbs of yoga.

What is the 8-fold Path of Yoga?

When studying yoga sutras, you will instantly discover that it comes with a collection of practices and observances designed to guide you on your entire spiritual journey. This specific collection of practices is classified as the 8-fold path of yoga or 8 limbs of yoga. Here they are:

Yamas

Yamas is the first stage of the eight-fold path. It encompasses all the ethical rules practiced in Hinduism, and you can view these rules as moral codes or imperatives. As a social behavior, it encompasses the way you treat others, and the world surrounding you.

To get past this stage successfully, mastering the following five Yamas categorized as your moral principles is important.

> • Satya, which is about truthfulness – This means staying away from falsehood or anything that takes you away from the truth. To master this Yama, tell no lies. One example of deviating from Satya is cheating or lying about your income tax.

> • Ahimsa, which tackles non-violence – It trains you to stop harming all creatures in deeds and in thoughts. This Yama tolerates no form of violence, whether it is in action, words, or thoughts.

• Asteya, which focuses more on non-stealing – Means practicing the habit of not stealing or even intending to steal others' property through thoughts, speech, and action. Asteya does not just encompass material things. It also includes intangibles, like stealing your child's opportunity to learn independence and responsibility, which might happen if you stop him from doing something on his own.

• Brahmacharya, which is all about chastity, sexual restraint, and marital fidelity – No, this does not mean you should practice celibacy when you become a yogi. You are free to get married and build your own family. What this Yama means is to avoid too much self-absorption. Instead, your focus should be to dwell in the vastness, which means seeing the divinity in everything.

• Aparigraha (which tackles non-possessiveness and non-avarice) – By mastering this specific Yama, you can finally set yourself free from unnecessary hoarding and collecting, thereby letting go of your greed.

For instance, you must stop yourself from collecting more shoes or buying a car on a whim. Being in this stage also means letting go of your desire to monopolize conversations just because you want to be the center of attention. Live in simplicity and share everything, including your space, time, and silence, instead.

The practices and concepts included in this stage of yoga's 8-fold path are necessary for attaining the last stage, which is Samadhi. These moral codes restrain and prevent you from doing something that may hinder your personal growth.

For instance, a sutra brought up by Patanjali states that the habit of preventing yourself from injuring others or demonstrating violence can help you abandon enmity. Once it happens, you can perfect your outer and inner amity with all the people and things around you.

Niyama

This second stage of the 8-fold path of yoga encompasses those principles and practices you must live by to enjoy a happy and morally correct life. It covers a few virtuous observances and habits, and your duties, but it also highlights the action you must do towards the outside world.

It has the prefix "ni," the Sanskrit equivalent of within or inward. Getting into this stage requires mastering:

- Shaucha, which is all about practicing purity – It is attainable by practicing the first five Yamas, and can eradicate all your negative mental and physical states. This Niyama is also about keeping yourself, clothing, and surroundings clean. It requires treating your body with care and respect and ensuring that you nourish it with healthy and fresh foods.

- Santosha, which tackles contentment – This Niyama tackles the importance of finding genuine happiness with whom you are and what you currently have. Here, you must accept yourself, taking responsibility for your present circumstance, and finding genuine happiness by being in the moment.

- Tapas, which tackles discipline - It lets you hone critical and vital life skills, including persistence, self-discipline, and perseverance. To achieve that, cultivate discipline not only in your mind but also in body and speech. The main goal of building self-discipline is to have full control. It also directs your body and mind to reach higher spiritual purposes and aims.

- Svadhyaya, which involves the study of your own self and Vedas – This specific Niyama will teach you how to introspect your own speech, actions, and thoughts, and do a more thorough self-reflection.

• Ishvarapranidhana, which requires you to contemplate on Ishvara – helped by this Niyama, you can understand the supreme being or god and be familiar with your true self. You can also fully comprehend unchanging realities once you practice this Niyama.

Like Yamas, the yoga sutras of Patanjali also present ways to use each Niyama to achieve personal growth. Among the things you can cultivate within yourself are acceptance and contentment – both of which are instruments for genuine happiness – one that comes from within. With acceptance and contentment, it would be easier for you to stop your desires for all sources of worldly and material pleasures.

You can practice Niyama to travel even further along your path to becoming a yogi. It is necessary to build character throughout the process until you reach the final stage, Samadhi.

Asana

The third state is Asana. It focuses more on practicing physical yoga postures. It refers to the physical aspect, a vital step when trying to achieve freedom through yoga. Note that asana is not completely about cultivating a yogi's skill to do an impressive backbend, headstand, or any other complex poses. It specifically indicates the seat which is what you should take when practicing meditation.

Based on Patanjali's instructions, the only alignment you must practice for asana is a comfortable and steady posture. This means doing poses that are comfortable enough to prevent yourself from quivering.

When practicing various asanas or poses, remember that you can't classify a pose which triggers restlessness or pain as part of yoga. Also, according to yoga sutras, it is a requirement to practice proper spinal posture by keeping your head, chest, and neck erect every time you do sitting meditation. Your posture should be easy and steady.

Patanjali even compares the pose as resting similarly to a cosmic serpent who is calmly in the water of infinity. While some perceive practicing asana or postures as a form of workout or a method of staying fit, Patanjali, together with other ancient yogis, believed that it is still crucial in preparing one's body for meditation.

This is because sitting for a long period in contemplation requires a yogi to have a cooperative and supple body. It requires you to free your body from physical distractions, giving you full control of it as well as of your mind.

The main idea is always sitting comfortably. Try to avoid experiencing body pains and aches or any form of discomfort as such might distract you or cause restlessness. If you do that, you will be one step closer to attaining peace, happiness, and freedom through yoga.

Pranayama

This fourth stage of Ashtanga yoga, an essential requirement in reaching Samadhi, is about practicing breathing techniques. The goal is to learn how to breathe so you gain full control of your life force energy. Prana serves as the energy or life force, which you can see existing everywhere. It flows freely through proper breathing.

So, this stage is all about controlling your breath. It involves basic movements relevant to breathing, including inhalation, exhalation, and breath retention. By mastering proper breathing techniques, you can cultivate positive perceptions of things.

In Pranayama, it is necessary to abide by proper rhythmic patterns linked to deep and slow breathing. Practicing this stage is necessary for purification and the eradication of distractions from your mind. If you achieve that, you can easily concentrate and focus on your meditation sessions.

Various breathing techniques can change your mind in different ways. You can go for calming practices, such as the moon piercing breath (*Chandra Bhadana*), or stimulating ones, such as the shining skull cleansing breath (*Kapalabhati*).

Regardless of the breathing technique you've chosen to practice, it can still greatly contribute to changing your state of being positive. Just make sure to practice it while aiming to control your feelings or set yourself free from any negativities your mind habitually had.

Pratyahara

The next of Ashtanga yoga is Pratyahara. It is the fifth limb which is all about sensory transcendence or sense withdrawal. It is called Pratyahara from *Pratya*, which means to draw back or in or withdraw, and *Ahara*, which signifies anything you take in by yourself. Some examples are the different sounds, scents, and sounds taken in by your senses continuously.

In this specific stage, exert an effort to draw your awareness and consciousness from the outside stimuli and external world. It is necessary to direct your attention to what is internal.

Practicing Pratyahara lets you step back so you can look closely at yourself and reflect. That you need to withdraw from all your senses means you can observe your cravings in a more objective manner. That way, you can reflect on those unhealthy habits that might hinder your overall health and your inner growth.

Make it a point to practice this stage every time you meditate. Do it every time you perform breathing exercises or yoga poses, too. Basically, anytime you wish to direct your attention and focus internally is a chance to practice Pratyahara.

Cultivating a high level of focus and concentration may be extremely hard once you are already in your yoga room. It's true, especially if you have not mastered the art of withdrawing from your senses or getting rid of distractions. You can fight such a difficulty once you finally mastered Pratyahara.

When that happens, you will notice a subsequent improvement in your focus and concentration since nothing can distract you – even the smell of food outside or the sound of a mosquito flying around. The fact that *drawing in* means focusing on your breathing also means this limb directly relates to practicing Pranayama. It can also bring you much closer to the final stage, which is Samadhi.

Dharana

The next phase is *Dharana*, which literally means focused concentration. It comes from the Sanskrit words "Dha," which means maintaining or holding, and "Ana," which translates to something else or others. It has a strong and close relationship with the fourth and fifth limbs – the Pranayama and Pratyahara.

This stage encourages you to focus strongly on something. It requires you to withdraw from your senses so you can bring your attention to the ultimate point of concentration. Also, to draw in your senses, having intent, focus, and concentration is a must.

This sixth limb requires you to take to heart the concept popularized by Patanjali, which involves binding your thought in just a single place to attain complete concentration. The primary objective here is to keep your mind still, pushing all superfluous thoughts away but in a gentle and gradual manner.

You can achieve such stillness and concentration through various means, including focusing on your breath, candle gazing (*Tratak*), and visualization, all of which are the sixth limb's famous practices. Once you master Dharana, concentration becomes effortless. One sign indicating that you are successful in letting your mind achieve full concentration is the inability to sense passing time.

Dhyana

Dhyana, which is the seventh limb or stage of Ashtanga yoga, is all about contemplation and meditation. It refers to the flow of focus and concentration without getting disrupted or distracted by anything. You may think this stage is like Dharana since the sixth stage is also all about concentration, but remember that the two stages differ.

One differentiating angle is that Dharana focuses on one-pointed attention, while Dhyana is all about reaching the ultimate state of keen awareness without focusing on an object. During this seventh stage, you can already quiet your mind, giving you the stillness necessary in preventing any thought from creeping in.

Note that reaching this state is admirable as the whole process requires a lot of stamina and strength. While it is challenging to get into this important stage, avoid giving up. Remind yourself that yoga takes a lot of steps. It is a long process, so congratulate yourself once you finally hit this seventh limb.

An advantage of reaching this state is heightened awareness and oneness with the universe. It is a big leap towards reaching Samadhi, the ultimate state in the 8-fold path.

Samadhi

The last phase you must reach in the 8-fold path is *Samadhi,* a Sanskrit term that means joining, putting together, combining, trance, harmonious whole, and union. Upon reaching this last stage, expect to be finally one with the primary subject of meditation.

It lets you get to that spiritual state wherein you can encourage your mind to get fully absorbed in something, particularly something you intend to contemplate. This full absorption is the reason your mind loses its sense of identity in this specific stage.

As for Patanjali, he describes Samadhi as the last stage of Ashtanga yoga. He also views it as a state of ecstasy. In this state, you will discover a more profound and deeper connection to the divine, which means having a strong internal connection to all living things.

Once you realize that you are already in this state, you will immediately notice genuine peace. It can let you experience the pure bliss associated with your oneness with the universe.

Being the last stage, Samadhi is the ultimate goal of anyone who practices yoga. Note that if you pause and scrutinize what you truly want in life, you will suddenly realize your experience when you are fulfilled, free, and happy. It is a feeling that can overpower desires, wishes, and hopes. It is what Samadhi is aiming to fulfill.

Samadhi is necessary for successfully completing your yogic path, which can bring you to what you aspire for deep inside – peace and happiness. It is also worth pointing out this last stage of yoga is not something that you can buy or possess. In other words, you can't expect it to be a permanent state.

Meant only to be experienced, devote yourself to the practice, continues to be in this state for the long term. Patanjali's yoga sutras even indicate the importance of being completely ready by freeing yourself from any impressions, like unwanted habits, desires, aversion, and attachment.

Aim to cultivate a fully pure mind so you can keep this vital state for a long time. By keeping your mind pure, you can experience Samadhi and make it stick with you for a long time.

What to Expect from Ashtanga Yoga

To learn more about Ashtanga yoga, then your top priority should be mastering the eight limbs and making them a part of your life. The reason is that Ashtanga yoga will always be a physically strong and traditional form of yoga. It will always revolve around the principle of having to incorporate the eight limbs into your life.

This type of yoga also seems to work for anyone who is up for a challenge. The main reason is that Ashtanga allows you to sweat out and build your outer and inner strength. It can significantly increase your sense and focus for your body. It can also provide an excellent cardio workout as it involves swift movements.

Considering the eight limbs, you must go through; you can safely assume that Ashtanga yoga increases your awareness of your own body's flow and movement. Also, expect to have an improved sense of rhythm from this form of yoga. That it lets you move at your own level and the pace is also a big advantage. Just stick to following the 8-fold path until you reach the goal, which is Samadhi.

Chapter 3: Samadhi Pada: The Basics of Samadhi

Like what was indicated earlier, Samadhi is the ultimate stage you must reach to make the most out of yoga's eight-fold path. It is all about having a fixed mind for comprehending or understanding yourself. You can finally say you have reached Samadhi if your mind gets into that state.

Samadhi is also all about reaching a soundless level of breathlessness. It allows you to be in that state wherein you can experience genuine bliss with your higher consciousness level. With that, it would be easier to perceive the unique and individualized identity of the soul and cosmic spirit.

Note that yoga requires following a unique path when reaching Samadhi. It is different than the versions used by the Hindu and Buddhists. Such a path was discussed in the previous chapter, the eight-fold yoga path.

Getting into Samadhi shows you have finally united three vital aspects of meditation, namely the meditator, the actual act of meditation, and the specific object of meditation called God.

As the ultimate stage, you can consider it as the climax of every intellectual and spiritual activity. It also relates to Samadhi Pada, which is the first chapter of Patanjali's yoga sutras. Here, your focus will most likely be on honing your concentration.

Containing 51 sutras divided into several sections, expect to learn a lot of things in this chapter. Among these is the description of yoga, different kinds of thoughts, how to un-color thoughts, practice and non-attachment principles, different phases or stages of concentration, commitments and efforts, obstacles or challenges and solutions, and positive results from retaining your mind's stability.

Here are the 51 yoga sutras in Samadhi Padha (the 1st chapter) with their translations based on the Sanskrit words composing them. With the sutras divided into sections, you can understand them even better.

Yoga Descriptions (1.1 to 1.4)

Yoga Sutras - Sanskrit	Translation	Word References
1.1: अथ योगानुशासनम् - atha yoga-anuśāsanam	Now, the practice of yoga.	Atha - now, from this point on Yoga - yoga (see definition in Sutra 2) Anusasanam - instructions to the practice
1.2: योगश्चित्तवृत्तिनिरोध - yogaś-citta-vṛtti-nirodhaḥ	Yoga is stopping the mind or thoughts from making modifications.	Yogah - Yoga Chitta - mind stuff, thought Vritti - ripples, modifications Nirodhah - to stop
1.3: तदा द्रष्टुः स्वरूपेऽवस्थानम् - tadā draṣṭuḥ svarūpe-'vasthānam	At that time, the seer or spectator's true nature or own form reposes.	tada - then, at that time drashtuh - the seer, the spectator svarupe - own form, true nature avasthanam – reposes
1.4: वृत्ति सारूप्यमितरत्र - vṛtti sārūpyam-itaratra	Otherwise, the seer/spectator forms the modifications/ripples of the mind.	vritti - ripples, modifications sa - similar rupyam - form itharatra - otherwise

The first section of the Samadhi Pada is all about preparation. It prepares you to practice yoga as it describes it specifically. Remember that you can only sincerely start your pursuit towards achieving self-realization, which is vital in your life, if you set your ultimate goal on top of your priorities beginning today.

In Patanjali's yoga sutras, the first word you will see is Atha, a Sanskrit word meaning "now" (1.1). The word implies the preparation for the auspicious phase of commitment and desire to realization, which is the goal when practicing yoga. Atha is one of the first four yoga sutras that describe the practice in the first chapter, the Samadhi Pada.

The next three sutras also describe yoga. Yoga sutra 1.2, for instance, indicates how you can slowly move your focus and attention inward while going through all phases and levels of your being. It will let you achieve mastery as you move along the way. You will often experience that when meditating.

Yoga sutra 1.3 lets you rest in your true nature that usually goes beyond the mentioned levels. Reaching this realization is the center of consciousness, which is the real meaning of yoga.

In yoga sutra 1.4, the emphasis is on the way you may have entangled yourself with false identities frequently. With that, you can easily detect misidentification, which is the sleep cycle you must wake up from. Such an awakening to your own self is the ultimate meaning of yoga.

Witnessing and Un-coloring Your Thoughts (1.5 to 1.11)

Yoga Sutras - Sanskrit	Translation	Word References
1.5: वृत्तयः पञ्चतय्यः क्लिष्टाक्लिष्ट - vṛttayaḥ pañcatayyaḥ kliṣṭākliṣṭāḥ	Modifications are five-fold: misery and non-misery.	vrittayah - ripples, modifications pangchatayyah – five-fold klishta - misery, painful aklishta - non-misery, not painful
1.6: प्रमाण विपर्यय विकल्प निद्रा स्मृतय - pramāṇa viparyaya vikalpa nidrā smṛtayaḥ	Right knowledge, false idea (wrong notion), fictitious (imaginative) perception, sleep and memory.	pramaana - right knowledge viparyaya - wrong notion, false idea vikalpa - imagination, fictitious perception nidraa - sleep smritayah - memory
1.7: प्रत्यक्षानुमानाअगमाः प्रमाणानि - pratyakṣa-anumāna-āgamāḥ pramāṇāni	Right knowledge come from direct perception, logical reasoning or inference, and scriptures.	pratyaksa - direct perception anumaana - logical reasoning, inference aagamah - scriptures pramaanaani - right knowledge

1.8: विपर्ययो मिथ्याज्ञानमतद्रूप प्रतिष्ठम् - viparyayo mithyā-jñānam-atadrūpa pratiṣṭham	Misconception is the false knowledge not in the form of or differs from reality.	viparyayo - misconception, indiscrimination mithya - unreal jnanam - knowledge atadroopa - not in the form of pratishtham – not based on reality
1.9: शब्दज्ञानानुपाती वस्तुशून्यो विकल्प - śabda-jñāna-anupātī vastu-śūnyo vikalpaḥ	Vikalpa is the knowledge through sound without the object in reality.	shabda - sound jnana - knowledge anupati - follows vastu - object soonya - without, devoid vikalpah - fictitious perception
1.10: अभावप्रत्ययाअलम्बना तमोवृत्तिर्निद्र - abhāva-pratyaya-ālambanā tamo-vṛttir-nidra	Sleep is the modification wherein the mind rests on the darkness that lacks impressions.	abhava - non-existence pratyayaa - impressions alambanaa - support, rest tamo - void, inertia, darkness vritti - modification of mind nidraa - sleep
1.11: अनुभूतविषयासंप्रमोषः स्मृति - anu-bhūta-viṣaya-asaṁpramoṣaḥ smṛtiḥ	Memory is the modification which takes content from the experience that has not yet disappeared fully.	anuboota - from the experience vishaya - content asam - not fully pramosah - disappear smiriti - memory

After understanding what yoga means in the first four sutras, you can familiarize yourself with the actual process associated with attaining the goal of yoga, which is self-realization in sutras 1.5 to 1.11. These sutras will walk you through the different types of thoughts that might interfere with your progress and prevent you from reaching your goal.

Among the kinds of interfering mental impressions that might stop you from realizing your true self as indicated in this section of Samadhi Pada are:

- Knowing correctly

- Imagination

- Incorrect knowing

- Memory

- Deep sleep

In this specific section, you will discover ways to hone the first thought, knowing correctly. Also, be aware that these thoughts are Klishta (colored) or Aklishta (not colored). Simply observing whether your thoughts have or have no color is essential when undergoing balancing, calming, stabilizing, or purifying your mind. Doing so will make it possible for you to get into deeper meditation.

Witnessing and exploring the five different kinds of thoughts is also the key to learning how you can let their individual colors fade. It also informs you on how to take advantage of yoga meditation to achieve such a purpose. It slowly thins the veil of truth, which is necessary for experiencing your genuine and true self.

Witnessing and observing the actual color of your thought patterns is a useful practice of yoga. Fortunately, you can do it at any time of the day. It allows you to meditate in action or practice mindfulness, which can contribute to clarifying your clouded mind. With that, expect to go a lot deeper into the practice during the time you do the seated meditation.

Witnessing the color of your thoughts is not a complicated process. It just simply means identifying whether a thought, along with its emotion, is colored or not every time it arises. This section of the yoga sutras also requires you to figure out whether an action or decision is useful. By observing it and identifying if it is useful or not, you will have full complete control of your habits.

With un-coloring deep impressions and thoughts, remember that it comes in stages. When doing the un-coloring process, your goal is to stabilize your mind slowly and weaken the identified colorings along the process. After achieving that, you can get a glimpse of what is beyond your thought impressions and their individual colorings.

Practice and Non-attachment (1.12 to 1.16)

Yoga Sutras - Sanskrit	Translation	Word References
1.12: अभ्यासवैराग्याअभ्यां तन्निरोध - abhyāsa-vairāgya-ābhyāṁ tan-nirodhaḥ	Practice and dispassion control/stop the mind's modifications.	abhyasa - practice vairagya - dispassion abhyam - together tan - their nirodhah - stop, control
1.13: तत्र स्थितौ यत्नोऽभ्यास - tatra sthitau yatno-'bhyāsaḥ	Practice is the effort for the continuous maintenance of stopping modifications.	tatra - there sthitau - for the maintenance, situated yatna - efforts abhyasa - practice
1.14: स तु दीर्घकाल नैरन्तर्य सत्कारा असेवितो दृढभूमि - sa tu dīrghakāla nairantarya satkāra-ādara-āsevito dṛḍhabhūmiḥ	When observed constantly with devotion for a long time, it is firmly established.	sa tu - that too, but deergha - long kaala - period of time nairantarya - constant, permanently satkaara - with devotion, reverence asevito - adhered dridha - strongly based bhoomihi - earth, ground, basement

1.15: दृष्टानुश्रविकविषयवितृष्णस्य वशीकारसंज्ञा वैराग्यम् - dṛṣṭa-anuśravika-viṣaya-vitṛṣṇasya vaśīkāra-saṁjñā vairāgyam	Dispassion is the consciousness of mastery attained by controlling desires of objects whether seen or heard.	drishta - seen, perceived anushravika - heard, from scriptures vishaya - objects vitrishnnasya - who has control over desires vashikaara - mastery samjna - consciousness vairaagyam - dispassion
1.16: तत्परं पुरुषख्यातेः गुणवैतृष्ण्यम् - tatparaṁ puruṣa-khyāteḥ guṇa-vaitṛṣṇyam	The Supreme Purusha is realized by showing indifference or having no desire to the qualities of various nature's objects.	tat - that param - supreme purusa - the seer khyati - realization guna - qualities (sattva, rajo and tamo) vaitrsnyam - absence of desire

In this section of Samadhi Pada, you will discover two principles that serve as the core of yoga – Abhyasa, which means practice, and Vairagya, which means non-attachment. These are two vital principles because the whole system of yoga rests on them.

With this section, you can understand the significance of understanding the two mentioned principles. By doing so, you gain full control and mastery over your mind field and realize your true self. Here, practice means developing an attitude of persistence, requiring you to exert effort persistently to achieve and retain a state of tranquility and stability.

For you to be well-established in this principle, commit to exerting effort for a long time. As much as possible, do it taking no break. This stance will let the deeper practice unfold continuously, making it possible for it to go even deeper to your eternal core's direct experience.

Non-attachment is a principle, which serves as a vital companion of the practice. Cultivate it as it lets you set yourself free from all those that block you from achieving progress when doing yoga. Among those you can easily let go of once you master non-attachment is fear, false identities, and aversions – all of which may cloud your genuine self.

Practice and non-attachment work well together, with the former leading you to the right and proper path. The latter allows you to continue with your journey towards finding inner peace and happiness. It does so without the pleasures and pains you may encounter along the process. Such pleasures and pains might sidetrack you or divert your attention.

Slowly, you can expand your non-attachment until you reach the depth of your own Gunas (subtle building blocks) and that of the universe. Getting through this stage successfully will let you attain supreme non-attachment, which is also the key to bringing you closer to your ultimate goal of achieving final liberation.

Kinds of Concentration (1.17 to 1.18)

Yoga Sutras - Sanskrit	Translation	Word References
1.17: वितर्क विचारानन्दास्मिता रूपानुगमात् संप्रज्ञात - vitarka-vicāra-ānanda-asmitā-rupa-anugamāt-samprajñātaḥ	Samaadhi with consciousness happens in four forms: with reasoning, deliberation, happiness, and self-consciousness.	vitarka - reasoning, argumentation vichaara - discrimination, deliberation aananda - bliss, happiness asmitaa - self-consciousness rupa - form anugamaat - happen samprajnaatah - with consciousness
1.18: प्रत्यया भ्यास पूर्वः संस्कार शेषो ऽन्य - virāma-pratyaya-abhyāsa-pūrvaḥ samskāra-śeṣo-'nyaḥ	The other Samaadhi is the stoppage caused by consistent practice and retaining only the past impressions that did not manifest.	viraama - stopping, blocking pratyaya - caused by abhyaasa - consistent practice poorvah - past samskaara - impressions sesa - remain, leftovers anyah - other

After building the principles of practice and non-attachment, it is necessary to move inward based on the four stages or levels of concentration indicated in sutra 1.17. Progress into objectless concentration is stated in 1.18, too. Based on these sutras, you can view the different stages, levels, and classifications of concentration.

The first one is that requiring an object to focus or concentrate on. All objects of concentration will be any of the four stages, categories, or levels, namely:

> • **Savitarka** - This stage involves concentrating on a gross object while letting your mind do other activities. It lets you meditate on sensory awareness, gross level of breath, visualized objects, mantra syllables, and attitudes.

> • **Savichara** - In this stage, you can concentrate on subtle objects after leaving behind the gross ones. Some examples of your meditation, non-attachment, and inquiry objects once you reach this stage of concentration are subtleties of energy, the mind, senses, and matter.

> • **Sananda** - This stage emphasizes on the subtler condition of bliss when you meditate. You will also notice that your concentration is already free of subtle and gross impressions in the previous stages once you get into Sananda.

> • **Sasmita** - This form of concentration targets *I-ness* - the subtlest of them all. It relates to the *I* behind - or the witness to - your other experiences.

Aside from the four mentioned stages of concentration with an object, there is also what we call an *objectless concentration*. It requires you to release all the objects from your attention or focus.

Commitments and Efforts (1.19 to 1.22)

Yoga Sutras - Sanskrit	Translation	Word References
1.19: भव प्रत्ययो विदेह प्रकृति लयानाम् - bhava-pratyayo videha-prakṛti-layānām	For demi-gods or those with bodiless consciousness and those merged with nature, asamprajnata happens by birth.	bhava - become, manifest, the world pratyaya - cause, caused by videha - those with bodiless consciousness prakrti - nature layaanaam - merged with
1.20: श्रद्धावीर्यस्मृतिसमाधिप्रज्ञापूर्वक इतरेषाम् - śraddhā-vīrya-smṛti samādhi-prajñā-pūrvaka itareṣām	For others, dedication, determination, mindfulness, samadhi and self-awareness leads to asamprajnata.	sraddha - dedication virya – power with determination, willpower smrti – memory, mindfulness samaadhi – the advanced stage of meditation prajna – consciousness, awareness of being poorvaka – happens before itaresaam – others
1.21: तीव्रसंवेगानामासन्न - tīvra-saṁvegānām-āsannaḥ	The intense passion towards the practice and dispassion leads to the proximity of asamprajnata samaadhi.	Theevra – intensive, vigorous samvega – impulse, enthusiasm aasannah – bring to the proximity

		Mridu - tender, mild
1.22: मृदुमध्याधिमात्रत्वात् ततोऽपि विशेषः - mṛdu-madhya-adhimātratvāt-tato'pi viśeṣaḥ	The intense passion towards dispassion and practice again is classified into three kinds - mild, moderate and strong.	madhya - moderate
		adhimaatra - extreme, strong, intense
		tataah - from these
		api - also
		viseshah - specialty, kinds, types

Commitments and effort are where you need to focus on in yoga sutras 1.19 to 1.22. This section covers two types of aspirants capable of reaching the goal of practicing yoga. The first one is advanced, which is anyone who made a significant advancement in the way he/she lives his/her life in the past and now easily attains Samadhi.

The second one encompasses the other aspirants. A lot of those who practice yoga fall under this second type, requiring them to cultivate the five different kinds of commitment and effort. Here they are:

Sraddha

This commitment and effort is all about having the faith and belief you are taking and moving in the proper path or right direction. It refers to the internal feeling of certainty - one that assures you that you are pushing yourself to move on the correct path.

Even if you are still unaware of how your journey will unfold, have that inner intuition you are steadily walking towards your ultimate life goals. Building this type of effort, but does not mean cultivating blind faith. Testing ideas in your internal laboratory is even more essential. It lets you discover which idea will work for you based on your direct experiences.

For instance, if you practiced diaphragmatic breathing and breath awareness and discovered that both helped you calm and quiet your mind, it would be a direct experience that proves how doing such breathing exercises can produce similar positive results, like mental calm and quietness.

Veerya/Virya

It refers to your ego's positive energy, which acts as strong support of the faith you have cultivated. The energy of Virya you can develop here will give you the power and sense of knowing exactly what you should do. Strongly acting based on what you know as the right or correct path points to Virya.

However, weakness and uncertainty that may cause you to take little action are signs that your Virya is lacking. Develop this positive energy to let you attain your goals in yoga.

Smriti

This effort encompasses mindfulness and memory. It is all about honing constant mindfulness associated with treading the right path and having memories of the steps you have taken along the way.

But you can't classify the memory you cultivated here as a negative mental obsession. It is a gentle yet persistent awareness of your unique life goals, your strong belief and faith in the journey and decision to dedicate and commit a lot of your energy throughout the process. Smriti also requires you to practice mindfulness, particularly on inner processes.

Samadhi

Samadhi, in this section of the yoga sutra, refers to the commitment to move systematically through various stages and levels. It also requires using your already-developed skills of attention as tools to discriminate different kinds of ignorance. Moreover, it requires committing to remember the process of moving systematically through the fine levels of your being.

Prajna

This refers to the higher wisdom derived from discrimination. This wisdom is what you should seek for assiduously through introspection using the razor-sharp tool called Samadhi. The commitment and effort to pursue higher wisdom is further highlighted in the second and third chapters of the yoga sutras.

Now that you know the five kinds of effort and commitment, you must focus on cultivating them. Remind yourself of these five forms you have cultivated as such is the key to understanding yoga practices. Your knowledge will also inspire you to follow through on performing the exact practices recommended throughout Patanjali's yoga sutras.

AUM or OM Contemplation (1.23-1.29)

Yoga Sutras - Sanskrit	Translation	Word References
1.23: ईश्वरप्रणिधानाद्वा - īśvara-praṇidhānād-vā	Worshipping God also lets you attain Samaadhi.	Isvara - God Pranidhaanaat - worship vaa - also
1.24: क्लेशकर्मविपाकाशयैरपरामृष्टः पुरुषविशेष ईश्वर - kleśa karma vipāka-āśayaiḥ-aparāmṛṣṭaḥ puruṣa-viśeṣa īśvaraḥ	God is a special Being free of afflictions, actions, fruits of actions, and impressions	kleśa - afflictions karma - actions, causes vipāka - the fruits of actions, effects āśayaiḥ - resting place, impressions aparāmṛṣṭaḥ - untouched puruṣa - Self, Atman, Consciousness, Spirit viśeṣa - special īśvaraḥ - God
1.25: तत्र निरतिशयं सर्वज्ञबीजम् - tatra niratiśayaṁ sarvajña-bījam	In God, the seed of omniscience is at a superior level.	tatra - in that (special Being) niratiśayaṁ - unsurpassed, ever superior sarvajña - all knowing, omniscience bījam - seed

1.26: स पूर्वेषाम् अपि गुरुः कालेनानवच्छेदात्॥२६ - sa pūrveṣām-api-guruḥ kālena-anavacchedāt	Not being interrupted or limited by time, He is also the master of the ancients.	sa - He pūrveṣām - earlier api - too, even, also guru - master kālena - by time anavacchedāt - without interruption
1.27: तस्य वाचक् प्रिव् - tasya vācakaḥ praṇavaḥ	His word is Pranava.	tasya - His vācakaḥ - word, term Pranava - Om, AUM
1.28: तज्जप स्तदर्थभावनम् - taj-japaḥ tad-artha-bhāvanam	The continuous chant of Pranava with the absorption on its meaning is the means to attain Samadhi.	tad - its japa - chant tad - its artha - meaning bhāvanam - absorption
1.29: ततः प्रत्यक्चेतनाधिगमोऽप्यन्तरायाभावश्च - tataḥ pratyak-cetana-adhigamo-'py-antarāya-abhavaś-ca	By this, reaching samadhi, and clearing obstacles, too is possible.	tata - by this pratyak - individual cetana - consciousness adhigama- reaching api - also antarāya - obstacles abhavaś - clear ca - too

In this specific section of the Samadhi Pada, you will discover that most consider OM (AUM) as a direct path. Here, remember the sound vibration produced by OM (AUM) together with the deep emotion or feeling for its represented meanings.

By doing that, it is possible to realize your unique self and remove any obstacle that often blocks such a realization. This practice is like a shortcut, as it goes directly to the process's heart. It also involves taking you to a direct path inward by piercing your consciousness's different levels systematically.

It is necessary to do this process with dedication and sincerity so you can reach your untainted source of creativity and your pure consciousness – both of which are represented by AUM. This consciousness also composes your seed of omniscience, the ultimate source of all ancient sages' teachings.

To produce the best effect, remember the sound and vibration of AUM. Connect it with deep emotions and feelings for whatever it represents.

Obstacles or Challenges and Solutions (1.30 to 1.32)

Yoga Sutras - Sanskrit	Translation	Word References
1.30: व्याधि स्त्यान संशय प्रमादालस्याविरति भ्रान्तिदर्शनालब्ध भूमिकत्वानवस्थितत्वानि चित्तविक्षेपास्तेऽन्तराया - vyādhi styāna saṁśaya pramāda-ālasya-avirati bhrāntidarśana-alabdha-bhūmikatva-anavasthitatvāni citta-vikṣepāḥ te antarāyāḥ	The obstacles of Samadhi result from distractions of the mind caused by disease, dullness, doubt, negligence, sloth, overindulgence, imaginary ideation, inability to reach the milestone and instability.	vyādhi - disease styāna - rigidity, dullness saṁśaya - doubt pramāda - negligence ālasya - sloth avirati - overindulgence bhrāntidarśana - imaginary ideation alabdha - inability to obtain bhūmikatva - ground, milestone anavasthitatvāni - instability citta-vikṣepāḥ - distractions of mind te - these are antarāyāḥ - obstacles

1.31: दुःख दौर्मनस्याङ्गमेजयत्व श्वासप्रश्वासा विक्षेप सहभुव - duḥkha-daurmanasya-aṅgamejayatva-śvāsapraśvāsāḥ vikṣepa sahabhuvaḥ	The simultaneous experience along with the distractions are the pain, mental agitation, tremor of limbs and irregular breathing.	duḥkha - pain, suffering daurmanasya - mental agitation, imbalance aṅgamejayatva - tremor of limbs śvāsa praśvāsāḥ - irregular breathing vikṣepa - distractions sahabhuvaḥ - simultaneous experience
1.32: तत्प्रतिषेधार्थमेकतत्त्वाभ्यास - tat-pratiṣedha-artham-eka-tattva-abhyāsaḥ	To counteract this, the practice for a single subject is proposed.	tat - that pratiṣedha - counteract artham - for eka - single tattva - subject abhyāsaḥ - practice

This section leads to the immediate realization there will always be challenges and obstacles along the way. The obstacles could be predictable, taking place during your inner journey with a few other consequences resulting from them.

Dealing with them can be challenging, but the sutras can also make you feel comfortable knowing that such obstacles are predictable and natural parts of your journey. This knowledge can help you maintain your conviction and faith you can achieve your final goal.

In this section, the yoga sutras highlight the predictable challenges or obstacles you may encounter, including doubt, dullness, illness or disease, cravings, instability, failure, misperceptions, laziness, and negligence. It also lets you know the companions to these challenges or obstacles, including physical and mental pain, irregular breath, frustration, sadness, and unsteadiness of the physical body.

In this section, a yoga sutra, specifically 1.32, also indicated the solution, which is the mind's one-pointedness. It is the only underlying principle, which works as an antidote for all the mentioned obstacles and consequences.

You can practice it in many forms, but you can still expect the principle behind it to be uniform. One way to practice it is to remind yourself repeatedly about a single object or one aspect of the truth. It could be an object or those suggested in the sutras in the next section.

Keeping the Mind Clear and Stable (1.33 to 1.39)

Yoga Sutras - Sanskrit	Translation	Word References
1.33: मैत्रीकरुणामुदितोपेक्षणां सुखदुःखपुण्यापुण्यविषयाणां भावनातश्चित्तप्रसादनम्॥३३॥ - maitrī karuṇā mudito-pekṣāṇāṁ-sukha-duḥkha puṇya-apuṇya-viṣayāṇāṁ bhāvanātaḥ citta-prasādanam	The mind becomes purified by practicing friendship over wellness, kindness over suffering, pleasure over virtuosity and indifference over immorality.	maitrī - friendship karuṇā - kindness mudita - merry upekṣāṇāṁ - indifference sukha - wellness duḥkha - suffering puṇya - virtuous apuṇya - immoral viṣayāṇāṁ - matters bhāvanātaḥ - practiced citta - mind prasādanam - purified
1.34: प्रच्छर्दनविधारणाभ्यां वा प्राणस्य॥३४॥ - pracchardana-vidhāraṇa-ābhyāṁ vā prāṇasya ॥34॥	It is also attainable by practicing gradual nasal expiration and control of breath.	pracchardana - gradual nasal expiration vidhāraṇa - control ābhyāṁ - together vā - also prāṇasya - prana

1.35: विषयवती वा प्रवृत्तिरुत्पन्ना मनसः स्थितिनिबन्धिनी॥३५॥ - viṣayavatī vā pravṛtti-rutpannā manasaḥ sthiti nibandhinī	By fixing the mind on a single modification generated by sensory objects, it is possible to attain the fastness of mind.	viṣayavatī - impressions stimulated by objects vā - also pravṛtti - modifications utpannā - generate manasaḥ - mental sthiti - stability nibandhinī - fastness, the state of being fixed/bound
1.36: विशोका वा ज्योतिष्मती ॥३६॥ - viśokā vā jyotiṣmatī ॥36॥	Also, by the sorrowless and luminosity of the mind.	viśokā - devoid of sorrow, pain vā - also jyotiṣmatī - luminosity of the mind
1.37: वीतरागविषयं वा चित्तम् ॥३७॥ - vītarāga viṣayam vā cittam ॥37॥	Also, by meditation without attachment to sensory objects.	Vītarāga - without attachment viṣayam - sensory object(s) vā - also cittam - the mind stuff

1.38: स्वप्ननिद्राज्ञानालम्बनं वा ॥३८॥ - svapna-nidrā jñāna-ālambanam vā ॥38॥	Also, by the basis of the wisdom acquired during dream and sleep.	svapna - dream nidrā - sleep jñāna - wisdom, knowledge, experience ālambanam - basis vā - also
1.39: यथाभिमतध्यानाद्व ॥३९॥ - yathā-abhimata-dhyānād-vā ॥39॥	Also, by meditating on an object that pleases one.	yathā - that which abhimata - pleasing to one dhyānād - by meditation vā - also

Mental clarity and stability are necessary if you want to experience Samadhi or subtler meditations. In this case, this section of the yoga sutras can be a big help to you. Here, you will learn four important attitudes that will provide the clarity and stability of the mind you are trying to achieve.

For instance, you will discover four vital qualities or attitudes towards people, such as lovingness or friendliness, support or compassion, neutrality or acceptance, and goodwill or happiness. Each mentioned attitude is already a form of meditation. You need to cultivate the four positive attitudes so you can counteract the negative.

The goal here is to deal with people in a way that the positive attitudes you have cultivated will reign. For instance, you need to develop an attitude of kindness and friendliness when you think of people or whenever you are with them.

It also requires you to be more mindful and conscious of your mind's negative tendency so that you can promote only the useful and positive. One advantage of making such positivity reign is that it promotes stability while giving your mind the calmness and inner peace it deserves.

The yoga sutras in this section also offer reliable suggestions for improving and retaining your focus. In yoga sutras 1.34 to 1.38, you will discover a few suggestions of objects where you can focus your attention to, including sensation, a stream of the mind, inner luminosity, breath awareness, and stable mind contemplation.

The last sutra in this section (1.39) recommends practicing one-pointedness on anything you discovered as useful and pleasing. Never skip any of the recommendations in this section to make sure that you will not end up fighting with your mind instead of giving it the stability and clarity it needs.

Results of Keeping the Mind Stable (1.40 to 1.51)

Yoga Sutras - Sanskrit	Translation	Word References
1.40: परमाणु परममहत्त्वान्तोऽस्य वशीकारः ॥४०॥ - paramāṇu parama-mahattva-anto-'sya vaśīkāraḥ ॥40॥	By these practices, it is possible to attain mastery, which extends from the smallest atom to an object of extreme magnitude.	paramāṇu - extremely small atom parama-mahattva - extreme magnitude anta - as the end asya - belong to vaśīkāraḥ - mastery
1.41: क्षीणवृत्तेरभिजातस्येव मणेर्ग्रहीतृग्रहणग्राह्येषु तत्स्थतदञ्जनतासमापत्तिः ॥४१॥ - kṣīṇa-vṛtter-abhijātasy-eva maṇer-grahītṛ-grahaṇa-grāhyeṣu tatstha-tadañjanatā samāpattiḥ ॥41॥	The crystal-clear mind with controlled-modifications and stabilized to reflect the color of meditator, meditation and the object meditated appears as equal to them.	kṣīṇa - weakened iva - like grahaṇa - the act of perceiving vṛtti - modifications maṇeh - crystal grāhyeṣu - object perceived tad-añjanatā - taking the color of that abhijātasya - purifies grahītṛ - one who perceives tat-stha - stabilizing on that samāpattiḥ - become similar to

1.42: तत्र शब्दार्थज्ञानविकल्पैः संकीर्णा सवितर्का समापत्तिः ॥४२॥ - tatra śabdārtha-jñāna-vikalpaiḥ saṁkīrṇā savitarkā samāpattiḥ ॥42॥	Among the achieved balances of the mind, modifications regarding the choices of the word, its meaning and concept are linked to Samadhi with deliberation.	tatra - in there, among these śabda - sound artha - meaning vikalpah - with choices jñāna - wisdom, concept saṁkīrṇā - mingled with savitarkā - with deliberation samāpattiḥ - Samadhi, engrossment
1.43: स्मृतिपरिशुद्धौ स्वरूपशून्येवार्थमात्रनिर्भासा निर्वितर्का ॥४३॥ - smṛti-pariśuddhau svarūpa-śūnyeva-arthamātra-nirbhāsā nirvitarkā ॥43॥	When clearing the memory, the mind sheds lights only on the object's meaning and appears as if it lost its own form. This is Nirvitarka Samadhi, the Samadhi without discrimination.	smṛti - memory pariśuddhau - on purification iva - as it is śūnya - devoid of mātra - alone nirbhāsā - radiance svarūpa - own form artha - meaning nirvitarkā - without discrimination

1.44: एतयैव सविचारा निर्विचारा च सूक्ष्मविषया व्याख्याता ॥४४॥ - etayaiva savicārā nirvicārā cha sūkṣma-viṣaya vyākhyātā ॥44॥	By this, deliberative and non-deliberative thoughts regarding subtle things are explained.	etaya - by this eva - also nirvicārā - devoid of deliberative thoughts savicārā - with deliberative thoughts cha - and sūkṣma-viṣaya - subtle things vyākhyātā - explained
1.45: सूक्ष्मविषयत्वं चालिङ्गपर्यवसानम् ॥४५॥ - sūkṣma-viṣayatvam-ca-aliṅga paryavasānam ॥45॥	The subtlety pertains to objects ends with its unmanifested prime state.	sūkṣma - subtlety viṣayatvam - pertains to objects cha - and aliṅga - unmanifested state paryavasānam - ends there
1.46: ता एव सबीजः समाधिः ॥४६॥ - tā eva sabījas-samādhiḥ ॥46॥	These are only Samadhis with seed.	tā- - these, they eva - only sabīja - with seed samādhi - samadhi
1.47: निर्विचारवैशारद्येऽध्यात्मप्रसादः ॥४७॥ - nirvicāra-vaiśāradye-'dhyātma-prasādaḥ ॥47॥	The continuous flow of Nirvichara Samadhi results in the prevalence of clarity of Atman.	nirvicāra - Nirvichara Samadhi vaiśāradye - the flow without break adhyātma - pertains to Atman prasādaḥ - clarity

1.48: ऋतम्भरा तत्र प्रज्ञा॥ - ṛtaṁbharā tatra prajñā ॥48॥	That is the consciousness filled with truth.	ṛtaṁbharā - filled with truth, tatra - therein prajñā - consciousness
1.49: श्रुतानुमानप्रज्ञाभ्यामन्यविषया विशेषार्थत्वात्॥४९॥ - śruta-anumāna-prajñā-abhyām-anya-viṣayā viśeṣa-arthatvāt ॥49॥	The consciousness by testimony and inference is different from the consciousness of Nirvichara, because in Nirvichara, the consciousness pertains to the specific particulars of the objects.	śruta - heard, testimony anya - different anumāna - inference viṣayā - objects prajñā-abhyām - from that knowledge viśeṣa - specific to arthatvāt - significance, meaning
1.50: तज्जः संस्कारोऽन्यसंस्कारप्रतिबन्धी ॥५०॥ -	The impressions arise therefrom blocks the other latent impressions.	tajja - arise from saṁskāra - latent impressions anya - different, other pratibandhī - contradictory, obstruct

		tasyā - in that, of that
1.51: तस्यापि निरोधे सर्वनिरोधात्रिर्बीजः समाधिः ॥५१॥ - tasyāpi nirodhe sarva-nirodhān-nirbījaḥ samādhiḥ ॥51॥	When these latent impressions too are suppressed, it becomes Nir-Bija Samadhi, the seedless one.	sarva - all
		api - too
		nirodhāt - controls
		nirodhe - controlling
		nirbījaḥ - Seedless
		samādhiḥ - Samadhi

This section talks about how the mind eventually turns into a clear and transparent crystal upon finally stabilizing it reasonably. If that happens, expect yoga's deeper process to start. As a more transparent crystal, your mind will most likely work as a highly purified tool for subtle explorations. With that, your mind can explore a wide range of objects, no matter how small or large they are.

Also covered in this section of Samadhi are four meditation levels when trying to focus on a single object. You may experience such levels systematically until you reach that one wherein unmanifest matter occurs.

In Samadhi, it is necessary to restrain unrest totally. With that said, Patanjali states that it is only achievable through meditation, particularly by going through its different levels and dimensions. These levels ensure that you can completely subside from aversion and desires, promoting calmness from your mental fluctuations called Vrittis. These fluctuations serve as the direct consequences based on where your unrest comes from.

If left undealt with, such mental fluctuations may cause you to deal with a stirring body and restless mind. The different levels or stages of meditation can help you in that area. Here they are:

• **Samapatti** – This level or stage allows all things to appear as they are. It is also the time when you need to go into deep reflection. In this stage, observe your inclination towards coloring reality using your projections.

But one thing to remember is that those inclinations with a specific end targeted tend to diminish their main purpose or aim. As the one who is meditating, you will witness not only the projections content but also their aim. It is possible with the guidance of your aversion or desire.

When you are in this stage, expect the insight regarding the game played with reality to arise. The way you color it will also come out.

• **Sabjasamadhi** – Once you experience this insight and it slowly transcends the game, you will notice genuine peace arising. When that happens, you can consider yourself in the second stage, the Sabjasamadhi, otherwise referred to as absorption with a germ.

Your personality's conscious part is devoid of your projection tendencies. Still, it comes with attention, which is also an intention despite its emptiness. It is where real peace, as well as the commencement of wisdom, runs. Sabjasamadhi is, therefore a stage, which works effectively in burning your inclinations to the project.

• **Nirbijasamadhi** – The last phase is Nirbijasamadhi, which has absorption without germ as its translation. Here, you will notice zero tendencies to get yourself detached from yourself. You will also notice deep absorption taking place spontaneously and naturally.

One vital reminder to yourself once you reach this state is that at first, meditation is only possible if you have a certain aim – and that is dissolving projecting tendencies or inclinations. Doing so can contribute a lot in keeping your mental fluctuations still.

What makes them distinguishable from normal tendencies that are unconscious and spontaneous is that the art of meditating is often staged deliberately. This means that you are willing to be conscious when trying to get into the object that you want to concentrate on during meditation.

One advantage is that it aids in dissolving your projecting tendencies. The result is the improved ability to cultivate peace and detachment.

The problem is that the entire process may lead to the birth of a new goal or tendency called the process of transformation towards genuine peace. Note that you can only reach Samadhi if you detach yourself from all tendencies toward it. If you can successfully do that, you can finally say that you are in Nirbijasamadhi, the absorption without germ.

This process is natural since when the main source of unrest diminishes its power, you can expect to develop an inclination towards Samadhi. If you relate it to the sutras, it is possible to experience remarkable results as you can perceive the proper balance between two mind movements – the positive and negative fluctuations. It indicates the transition from being held captive to be in a state of peace without any inhibitions, referred to as Kaivalya.

What is so great about mastering these meditation levels is that they can bring you a lot closer to your goal when practicing yoga. For instance, meditations on subtle and gross objects will result in inner luminosity, purity, higher wisdom, and reduced impressions driving karma. It also lets you experience the objectless Samadhi indicated in yoga sutra 1.51.

Apart from that, you can retain the stability of your mind. It can hone your power to build stability on the tiniest and largest object, which is a sign that your mind is already under your control. Fortunately, having full control over your mind helps you turn it into a tool.

You can use it as an instrument in exploring subtle parts of your mind field. The fact that you can control your mind also clearly indicates you already have the power to train it. With that, you can surely use your mind as a tool in doing things you have never thought possible.

PART TWO: Stages of Samadhi

Chapter 4: Four Crucial Stages of Samadhi

Samadhi is the most enlightening and joyous state you can reach when practicing yoga. Many even consider this stage as the primary precursor of happiness and enlightenment. Remind yourself that everyone plays a vital role in the universe. Regardless of your beginnings, your role in the universe matters a lot.

Another reminder about Samadhi is that you can't consider it as just one state. As a matter of fact, it comes with a set of stages unfolding in progression. Each stage yields two results – knowledge and non-attachment. This means that while some say that a stage helped them experience knowledge directly, others also practice non-attachment regardless of the degree or severity.

As soon as you let yourself advance to Sadhana, you can expect the knowledge you have gained to become more profound. Having non-attachment because of your journey may cause it to have a lasting and deep effect on your mind, but remember that every stage requires months (even years) to complete. You may need to spend more time than you initially expected to achieve your goal or get into that state wherein your mind is completely stable.

The length of time it will take for you to get your desired results to differ significantly. It usually depends on how intense your desire is towards achieving liberation. You can also base it on your intent and the frequency of practicing yoga and meditation, as well as your mental impressions (samskaras), particularly those derived from meditating in your previous life.

Remember that you can also get into the ultimate stage of Samadhi by surrendering to God. Moreover, it is necessary to have a full experience of what each phase or stage of Samadhi can reveal. This means getting completely absorbed in every stage, then diminishing your interest and attraction for each one as soon as you are ready to move on to the next stage.

Another reminder is that you can only progress through each stage successfully if you are willing to undergo the purification process. Fortunately, by doing things correctly, each stage can lead to the purification of your mind. The result is a subtler mind, which works better in going deep into various cosmic existence levels. With that, achieving the next stage will be more manageable for you.

Different Stages of Samadhi

Just like what has been mentioned earlier, you can only successfully reach Samadhi if you go through all its stages. It basically has three to four stages, but there are also methods that you can implement to guarantee a more smooth-sailing journey.

The following are just four of the basic stages of Samadhi that you must be aware of:

Samprajnata Samadhi

Also called Savikalpa, this is the stage wherein you experience quietness and peacefulness every time you meditate. As it is still the first stage, you will notice your availability to the outer world, even with the peace and quiet you are experiencing.

You can be in this stage by sitting quietly and making a conscious effort to remove all the mental disturbances bugging you while meditating. In case you notice stimulus happening, try responding to it using your knowledge (Prajna). By successfully doing that, you can finally say that you have mastered this stage.

Another sign that you have successfully reached this stage is experiencing conditioned oneness. This means mastering the habit of making your soul a part of your infinite consciousness. The only thing that differentiates it from the other stages of Samadhi is it comes with challenges when preserving such an experience out of your meditation session.

In other words, you can only make it happen out of meditativeness. It lets you diminish your human consciousness for a brief amount of time. It is also in this state wherein you will notice how different the concepts of space and time are when compared to their material counterparts. Another reminder about this state is that it is not permanent. This means that you will still go back to your usual consciousness.

Asamprajnata Samadhi

Also referred to as Nirvikalpa, Asamprajnata Samadhi refers to that stage wherein you let yourself go a lot deeper. This means finally drawing yourself away from the outside world. This stage has more depth and means that any stimulus will no longer affect you.

One prominent thing that tends to exist naturally when you get into this state is empty and pure consciousness. It also greatly improves your self-awareness. You will also notice your mind taking in omnipotent and omniscient traits of the cosmic.

By getting into this stage without any hassle, especially when navigating the whole experience, you will most likely attain discriminative wisdom and mental purity. This state also allows letting go of all your attachments, making you as free and pure as possible.

Dharma Megha Samadhi

This third stage is higher than Asamprajnata. Also referred to as the cloud of virtue, you will instantly realize you reached this state once you finally diminished even your desire to achieve enlightenment or be more knowledgeable about everything. This state is something you can't gain by effort. You will notice it revealing on its own once all your efforts and desires are already dissolved.

Many also consider it as a divine gift – one that goes beyond what is relative and absolute. If you are no longer distracted by the yogic powers' temptations, then it is safe to say that your pure and absolute knowledge is already overpowering them. Such signifies that you have already reached that cloud of virtue. It indicates that you have experienced the bliss and liberation of the divine.

It also shows that you have finally removed all afflictions from various forms of karma, a sign that you are already free and now shining in your own glory. Once you reach this glorified state, expect to be able to see, hear, smell, touch, and taste even without using your eyes, ears, nose, skin, and tongue.

You will also notice that even your mere intentions are already capable of working miracles. The only thing that you must do is set your intention, and you will notice all things coming to fruition.

Kaivalya Samadhi

While some translations of the yoga sutras indicate the Dharma Megha as the last stage of Samadhi, remember that some translated versions still talk about Kaivalya. In these versions, Kaivalya is the ultimate stage you must get into if you want to experience what it feels like to achieve yoga's main goal.

Reaching this stage means that you have finally reached the final, eternal, and complete union with the eternal and real form. It also means being detached and isolated. It allows you to get into a state of relaxed solitude.

You can say that you have achieved this state successfully once you get detached from everything that affects your entire being. This means gaining independence from everything, including your relationships, attractions, birth and death cycle, aversions, and egoism.

It is also possible to reach this state by practicing yoga, cultivating discipline, and performing austerities. Another thing that can help you understand Kaivalya Samadhi even better is one part of Patanjali's yoga sutras, which talked about a yogi.

Here, the yogi reached Kaivalya after seeking independence from all possible and existing bonds and attachments. Being in the stage allowed him to get into absolute consciousness. One advantage of attaining this final stage successfully is that it lets you enjoy true enlightenment.

Just like the third stage, you will feel free and fearless when you get into Kaivalya. Though there are times when people perceive Kaivalya as annihilation or negation, it is still worth pointing out that it is the stage when you achieve complete awareness of everything around you.

10 Methods of Samadhi

Aside from the mentioned stages, it is also crucial to note the ten methods that you can use to get yourself into the ultimate goal, Samadhi. Remember that Samadhi means that your mind is already free. You are finally detached from everything, particularly those that harm you.

Set your mind free as it consists of a bundle of desires (Vasanas) and imagination or thoughts (Sankalpas). It is also full of your likes and dislikes. Annihilate everything attached to your mind, so you can finally free it. You can do that with the help of the following methods:

• **Vichara** - When trying to get into Samadhi, you may ask yourself how you can purify your mind and put it under your complete control. You will start asking yourself and reflecting on your ability to stop your mind's activities and annihilate all distractions, desires, and anything attached to it.

One way to control your mind and annihilate its bonds and attachments is to use Vichara. This involves inquiring about who you are exactly. Spend time reflecting on yourself and finding out who you genuinely are is the most efficient method for attaining Samadhi.

By knowing yourself, you can easily annihilate your mind. Individuals also refer to this method as Vedantic. It involves knowing yourself and realizing or discovering the unrealities of your mind using philosophical thinking.

• **Eradicating Your Ego** - Another effective method associated with attaining Samadhi is getting rid of your egoistic personality. You need to remove your ego. Remember that your ego acts as the seed that cultivates the tree of your mind. Having a huge ego means thinking mostly of yourself.

The problem with having this "I" thought is that it can lead to it becoming the source of everything that runs through your mind. You will notice your thoughts focusing only on yourself and thinking little of others.

Determine if you have such an egoistic personality. Delve deeper into the things penetrating your mind, and you will immediately realize how your egoism translates to airy nothing.

If that is the case, it is time to free yourself from your ego. It is the key to bringing yourself to your desired Samadhi. Your goal is to get into the peak of self-realization so you can finally diminish that cloud of ego.

• **Dispassion** - You can also take advantage of dispassion (Vairagya) when trying to annihilate the mind. As the name suggests, dispassion is about cultivating distaste for anything that pleasures your senses on a whim. You can do that by determining those things you can consider as defective in your sensual life.

Your goal when using this method is to realize how perishable objects are. Remind yourself that sensual pleasure is only illusory. It does not last that long. It is only momentary, so you need to avoid putting all your passion, interest, and desire into it. By mastering the habit of perishing your passion for things giving you sensual pleasure, you can bring yourself closer and closer to Samadhi.

• **Abhyasa** - Another highly effective method that you can implement to reach Samadhi is practice or Abhyasa. Implementing this method involves concentrating your mind only on Brahman. Ensure that your mind is steady when fixing it to Brahman, too. Also, remember that Abhyasa is a form of ceaseless meditation that will eventually lead you to Samadhi.

• **Non-Attachment** - You can also lead yourself towards Samadhi if you make it a habit to practice non-attachment or Asanga. One advantage of this method is that it is highly effective in destroying all attachments and bonds your mind has.

To make this method work, remove your mind from objects. It also requires adhering to the detach and attach principle. This means detaching your mind from objects then attaching it to the Lord. You should then do this step repeatedly. Remember that regardless of how essential you perceive your desires are, the strength and fire of Asanga or non-attachment can still destroy it.

• **Vasanakshaya** - Another method that will surely lead you to Samadhi is Vasanakshaya derived from Vasana, which means desire. This method requires you to renunciate your desires. The result would be the successful annihilation of your mind. In this method, remember that having a desire for pleasurable objects might cause you to be in bondage.

You need to give up this desire so that you can get into emancipation. While desire is a vital nature of the human mind, learn to let it go if you want to get the best results from this Vasanakshaya method, especially in terms of driving yourself to Samadhi.

• **Pranayama** - The next method of Samadhi recommended to those who wish to attain it is Pranayama. Remember that Prana's vibrations may result in the movements of your mind. As a matter of fact, such vibrations can cause your mind to have life.

By controlling your Prana, which is what Pranayama is all about, you can stop your mind from doing all those unnecessary activities and movements. The good news is that even if this method involves stopping your mind from doing unnecessary activities, it will still not destroy it to its roots, giving you peace of mind.

• **Control of Thoughts** - Reaching Samadhi is also possible by properly controlling your own thoughts. What you should do is avoid daydreaming or being caught up by your own imagination. Annihilate the mind by releasing it from imagined thoughts.

By removing imagination from your mind, you will no longer have to worry about being in a world of illusion. You can stay away from this world and stop your imagination completely, allowing you to enjoy the moment and what is real.

• **Balance and Equanimity** - The next method that will lead you to Samadhi requires letting balance and equanimity reign. You can do that if you renunciate your possessions from your mind. This method can also benefit you in the sense that it will let you understand how you can get into the state of Samadhi, wherein you can suspend your thoughts.

When that happens, expect to realize absolute and pure experience. Make it a point to attain equanimity, too, which is possible by balancing things (ex. finding the right balance of pleasure and pain).

• **Devotion and Service** - This last method also effectively annihilates your thoughts or anything that may be bugging your mind. To make this method work, focus more on devotion and prayer. Also, prioritize studying and offering service to the guru. With that, you can get eternal bliss and everlasting peace that will transcend to your mind, a key in making Samadhi a part of your life.

With the help of these methods, bringing the state of Samadhi to you will be a lot more manageable. To increase your chance of enjoying the happiness and peace that Samadhi can bring, let us talk about each of its stages in detail. Learn more about the three important stages in the succeeding chapters of this book.

Chapter 5: The First Stage: Savikalpa Samadhi

Savikalpa Samadhi is the famous first stage of Samadhi indicated in Patanjali's yoga sutras. This stage is all about deliberation, bliss, reflection, and I-am-ness. It requires setting yourself free from your ego and raising your awareness about the spirit that goes beyond your creation.

When that happens, you can expect your soul to develop the ability to absorb the spirit-wisdom's fire, roasting or destroying any seeds of inclinations bound by your body. In this stage, the soul acts as the meditator. It needs to unite with the actual state of meditation as well as the spirit of the object you are using for meditation.

This can prompt everything to become one. It also means merging the soul with the spirit. You do not have to worry about losing your identity along the process as it just involves expanding your soul into a spirit.

Once you get into this first stage of samadhi, expect your mind to have its consciousness only directed on the spirit inside. This means you will no longer be conscious of what is happening in the outside world. It would be as if putting your body in a trance while still having a consciousness completely perceptive of the bliss you are experiencing within.

Your mind will still be active, making it possible for you to notice and observe your attachments to worldly and bodily distractions. Despite that, this stage will still give you a glimpse of what genuine bliss is all about. You can perceive the experience as conditioned oneness, which will surely push you to move on to the next level.

Also, remember that Savikalpa Samadhi is not permanent, meaning you will still have to go back to your usual consciousness. This stage is also further divided into four, namely:

Sarvitarka Samadhi

Here, you can transform your thoughts regarding a certain object you are using for your meditation sessions through words. If you are already practicing meditation, then it is highly likely that you have already experienced this stage several times, though it is unnoticeable.

Note that because of the many things that your mind processes every day, you may not sense right away that you are already at this level. Still, it is important to remember that this phase is all about acquiring knowledge. In yogic philosophy, knowledge comes with a sense of differentiating real from what is not all the time.

Once you are in the Sarvitarka Samadhi, you can use words in transforming your thoughts about an object. You can also begin a dialogue referred to as Tarka. Furthermore, in this state, your mind will begin weighing things using complete awareness and determining which ones are worthwhile and useful during discussions.

Aside from that, your mind can completely focus on the physical object's gross aspect. In other words, you will be on your way towards learning or scrutinizing the object's inner secrets. You can understand all aspects related to an object during this stage, giving you complete knowledge about it that will be useful in your journey towards becoming a successful yogi.

Savichara Samadhi

The next phase, Savichara Samadhi, is described in Patanjali's sutras, specifically 1:44 to 1:45. Getting into this phase means that your mind is already moving beyond an object's exterior layers. In other words, you will be using an object as the main point of your focus when you are at this level. Here, you will notice your mind finally honing its ability to contemplate or discern the object's subtle aspects.

You will also start fully understanding its abstract qualities, like sound, beauty, redness, flavor, form, texture, or love. Savichara Samadhi is also that state, which involves subtle objects extending to Prakriti, which is the main source of every manifestation. As soon as you move deeper into this phase, cultivating a better understanding of the real nature of space and time will naturally follow.

Aside from that, you can improve your knowledge about the vital aspects of the cosmic mind. Your mind will begin experiencing and exploring the object's subtler level by alternating your awareness of the object's causal, temporal, and special aspects.

In time and with proper practice, you can finally transmit your awareness to a higher level. It lets you achieve that state wherein complete silence is noticeable. Thinking is still available during this stage, but it is highly likely that your mind has already and finally mastered the ability to stay still and quiet.

Sa-ananda Samadhi

This third stage is all about freeing your mind from the objective world, making it possible for you to go beyond your intellect. In other words, you will get the chance to experience extreme bliss by ceasing your thoughts and removing logic occurring inside.

Sa-ananda Samadhi no longer involves any reflection or reasoning. It solely focuses on making you experience the peace and tranquility of having a more settled mind. It allows you to cultivate a pure (sattvic) mind characterized by awareness, focusing only on its own happiness.

In this stage, you will be focusing more on the internal powers of your mind and your perception. With that kind of experience, it is no longer surprising to see a lot of people perceiving it as a genuinely blissful form of Samadhi filled with joyful tranquility and peace.

Sa-Asmita Samadhi

Sa-Asmita is the last stage/phase of Savitarka Samadhi. You can expect it to happen once you finally mastered the single-pointed state of consciousness, purifying your mind and penetrating deeper. In this last phase, you will realize that even the bliss you have acquired in the previous stage is finally gone. The only thing that remains is ego – the I AM or I-ness.

This stage also makes you aware of your individuality. It allows you to stay in the moment and remove your awareness of anything else. It is actually the ego-sense presented in the elemental form without any desire nor fear. With that said, many liken this phase to the cosmic consciousness popularized in the Shankara tradition.

It involves having a completely awake mind while still being fully aware that what is in the outer world is just material and insignificant. Also, it can finally raise your awareness of the bliss of divinity that is within yourself. You will notice your mind becoming more concentrated, making it possible for it to start accessing lesser yogic powers.

One important reminder, though, is that your ego remains in this stage. With that said, be extra cautious when it comes to using yogic powers. Avoid using them to fulfill your ambition, and greed as such may only harm and delay your progress spiritually. Make it a point to use such yogic powers only if your heart and motives are pure. By doing that, you can offer your service to humanity while letting your spiritual journey progress.

How Does Savikalpa Samadhi Work?

If you want to reach Savikalpa Samadhi successfully, then you can take advantage of the power of meditation. However, the whole process also involves understanding the specific things that might be stopping you from getting into this first and important stage of Samadhi.

In that case, one important reminder to yourself is that at an unconscious level, a level categorized as being one with your thoughts and thinking, it is safe to assume that your thoughts can turn you into a victim. The main reason behind it is that your emotions and thoughts have full control over you. They even tend to build your world. Each thought you have turns into your reality.

For instance, if you have negative thoughts, like not being good enough, then it is also highly likely for your personality to reflect or resonate with such a thought. Being the center of that thought, expect feelings of inadequacy, like you not good enough. It might lead to unhappiness and stress, especially if you start taking in that thought personally and turn it into your reality.

You will also notice a contraction taking place often characterized by the feeling of stress brought on by each thought that you tend to identify with yourself. You can prevent that from happening through meditation. With that, you can see meditation as one of the most highly recommended techniques for anyone who wishes to attain success when trying to experience the first stage of Samadhi, which is Savikalpa.

Every time you meditate, you can always choose to identify yourself with your negative thoughts or just release them. If you choose the latter, then you can just act as a witness, proving the existence of such a thought. Meditation can contribute a lot in raising your awareness about your thoughts.

With that, every time you think you are not good enough, you can immediately detect such negativity, which also promotes ease in letting it go. The whole idea behind this is to prevent yourself from holding on to such a thought. It can subsequently result in you not having to deal with negative thoughts that may ruin your personality. Not holding onto your negative thoughts also means that they will not become personal to you.

Instead, what will happen is that you will turn into a witness who is in his ideal state of mind and peace. It is what you must achieve when planning to reach Savikalpa Samadhi. To make this method work for you, commit not to hold on to your thoughts too much, especially the negative ones about yourself, as catching the thought's content will only have negative consequences.

Remember that your thoughts will develop on their own. During each meditation session that aims to bring you closer towards the ultimate phase of Samadhi, the goal is not to control thoughts in a way that the process supersedes that of controlling your brain. With that said, you can still let your thoughts come to you. Just make sure that you only watch them.

When it comes to meditating to attain this stage, honing your focus and attention should be your top priority. You should strengthen your focus during each meditation session as it is the key to becoming more aware each time a thought comes out. If that happens, you can just watch it or let it go.

Also, remember that your thoughts will arise and diminish on their own. Avoid grabbing them at all, especially for a long time, to prevent them from hampering your progress. Hone your awareness about your thoughts as soon as they arise and master the skill of letting such thoughts go immediately.

One advantage of this technique is that once you start progressing, you will also be able to master that skill of not grasping all your thoughts. You will start letting them pass through instead. It happens once you also reached that level of focus or attention, wherein you can instantly see your thoughts as soon as they arise.

You may have a difficult time doing this at first. Fortunately, it gets easier and easier with constant practice. Also, note that you can release the next thought with each thought you have successfully released, making yourself stay as a witness. Observe when witnessing is already natural for you, too, as it signals that you have naturally penetrated the Savikalpa stage.

One point to remember when getting into the witness consciousness phase is that you will notice all your judgmental thoughts about others disappearing. With that, expect to be able to experience the highest form of peace in this level of consciousness. You will start experiencing all things simply as they are.

It usually happens because all thoughts regarding yourself will also start to diminish, like what you are thinking about your job, friends, life, movie you just saw, among many others. Every thought about you, as well as the way you live your life, will diminish, making it possible for you to enjoy amazing dreamlike visions arising on their own. The fact that these visions are not related to your personal life is the reason why they tend to burn away, but in genuine happiness, peace, and bliss.

Such an experience will also let your feeling and desire remain as a person disappearing temporarily. You will no longer feel the entire sense of being your own and having a body. You can also let go of your mind, making it possible to experience only consciousness, bliss, and formless energy. You will notice everything taking place simply then dissolving and transforming into spiritual energy, which is the ultimate work of Savikalpa Samadhi.

Chapter 6: The Second Stage: Nirvikalpa Samadhi

The second stage of Samadhi, which is called Nirvikalpa Samadhi, is all about reaching that meditative state that will give you an unforgettable experience of complete bliss and absorption. It lets you get into a higher state or level of awareness characterized by the successful elimination of ego and samskaras from your life and replacing them with only consciousness.

From Sanskrit, you can easily translate Nirvikalpa into the term "not wavering." This translation highlights the fact that Nirvikalpa Samadhi can be classified as a steady and sustained state. One thing to note about this state is that it is only usually attainable by those practitioners in more advanced stages. They include those who already achieved progress from the past stages, like those related to concentration (Dharana) and meditation (Dhyana).

Most spiritual masters can stay in this specific state for several hours. There are even masters who can stay in it for days. This can greatly benefit you as most say that being in Nirvikalpa Samadhi for up to eighteen to twenty-one days can help in enabling higher levels of Samadhi, particularly that state wherein you can let your consciousness leave your physical body permanently.

Unlike Savikalpa Samadhi, wherein you can keep your thoughts, though those do not impact you, Nirvikalpa involves merging your mental activities with yourself. This results in total and complete absorption, making it impossible for you to distinguish the knower, the known object, and the specific act linked to knowing.

Once you get into Nirvikalpa, expect your ego, and your samskaras that refer to your emotional or mental impressions, to dissolve. This can lead to having only your pure consciousness staying with you.

Here, you can unite with the Divine since you will be one. It allows you to merge your individual self, referred to as Atman, and your universal consciousness referred to as Brahman. With that, it is no longer surprising to see practitioners viewing Nirvikalpa as a stage of limitless bliss, genuine ecstasy, or oneness.

How to Get into Nirvikalpa Samadhi

If you want to get into Nirvikalpa Samadhi, which is also otherwise referred to as Asamprajnata Samadhi, then take note that there are also a few states that you must go through. Among the states you will experience when trying to reach this second stage of Samadhi is:

Nirvichara

In this stage, you will get to experience a genuine one-pointed focus and concentration. Here, even subtle thoughts are no longer existing. It transcends perceptual limitations linked to space and time. The fact that this state gets rid of your thoughts is the reason why some perceive it as samadhi without reflection.

Nirvichara is an important stage before reaching Nirvikalpa Samadhi. You must go through it if you want to strengthen your attention and turn yourself into a sane and wise person. Being in this stage also contributes to you gaining a much better understanding of your real identity and value. It helps you turn yourself into an instrument of divine love, which embodies pure love.

Nirvitarka

You can also reach Nirvikalpa samadhi by going through Nirvitarka, a state that allows you to encounter a suspension on the mental alterations of artha, shabda, and jñana. If you are still unfamiliar with the three mentioned terms, then here are their definitions:

- **Artha** - The recalled image or physical form of a certain object you see in the outer world.

- **Shabda** - Refers to the name or sound that you can use to communicate the object's identity to others.

- **Jñana** – Cultural or personal details about the purpose, function, or nature of such an object.

Once you get into Nirvitarka, expect these three to be suspended from your mind. Being the less real parts, jnana and shabda will also most likely fall away completely. Your mind will then be absorbed only in artha, though its full awareness that it is the knower will get diminished eventually.

In other words, Nirvitarka Samadhi is capable of temporarily transcending your memory of cultural and personal projections regarding the nature of the specific object you are focusing on. These projects include the object's identifying word or sound based on the practitioner's language and the accumulated personal insights and cultural knowledge derived from it.

Once that happens, you will notice your mind getting immersed only on artha as it does not only encompass the physical form's image but its related feeling, essence, and function, as well. It is possible to reveal all these elements using the single-pointed absorption of your mind.

Once your mind delves deeply into the object's artha, its gross form has the chance of transcending. You will also notice the object's subtle underlay getting revealed. With that, you get the chance to bring yourself to a state wherein you have better control over your ideas and mind and your dialogues and intellect.

Nirvitarka Samadhi can finally get you in that state wherein you were able to transcend whatever you remember about the object's nature temporarily.

Ananda to Asmita

You will also most likely go through Ananda to Asmita at the specific time you intend to reach Nirvikalpa Samadhi successfully. Ananda can be described as your consciousness of patterns among various paradigms. It involves pondering more on patterns instead of paradigm. From Ananda, you will most likely get into Asmita, which refers to the consciousness of being one.

Once you reach Asmita, you can no longer find any distinction on the few phases of awareness on your consciousness. In simpler terms, Asmita is all about the consciousness of wholeness. It lets you get into that specific level of consciousness, which many consider as omniscient when linked to the world of becoming while still being non-essential when compared to Kaivalya. It would be as if you are a huge fish in a small pond that mainly focuses on relative existence.

Getting into Asmita can also make you realize that even if you set aside all your false thoughts, desires, and identity during meditation, you will still notice a sense of I-ness being left behind. It is a sign that you have the veil of Asmita. The good news is that you can take advantage of this feeling by making it an object of focus during meditation. Asmita can even guide you towards reaching the most coveted stage in yoga, which is Samadhi.

What you must do is to direct your focus and attention to Asmita while standing alone. By doing that, you can eventually cause it to lose its color and set it aside. It somewhat proves that Asmita is one of those objects that you can use for meditating.

Also, it is crucial to note that all objects are constructed from Prakriti. It shows that even Asmita, which is the finest veil linked to individuality, is constructed from Prakriti, a delicate matter of manifestation. It is advisable to set aside all forms of Prakriti, so you can experience consciousness (Purusha) as it rests on true nature.

During the regular meditation practice, you will also notice the concepts revolving around Asmita swimming around your awareness. It will even become a vital component of your constant self-awareness.

Your full awareness of Asmita will also positively affect you in a way that it can raise the frequency of your use of such words in your usual vocabulary, especially when it comes to expressing yourself. With that, you will most likely discover the relationship of Smita to other processes, insights, and concepts. You will eventually learn how all the relevant concepts dance together, making it possible for you to have a guide towards understanding everything about them and beyond.

The reason behind it is that as you gain more self-awareness, you will also realize that all your observations do not define who you are in reality. In other words, you can never consider yourself an Asmita. Instead, you are someone capable of witnessing each concept. It makes it truly necessary to transcend Asmita and remove your attachment to it as much as possible.

Asmita to Nirbija Samadhi

Since you need to transcend Asmita and practice non-attachment to it, you must train yourself to get past through it and attain the level of Nirbija Samadhi. This concept makes use of the Sanskrit term, Nirbija, which means without seed. This specific level is considered as the highest since everyone can perceive it as the superconscious state linked to enlightenment.

Once you get into this level, you will notice your mind not containing any thoughts. What it contains, instead, would be pure awareness and consciousness. In Nirbija Samadhi, you get the chance to be one with your supreme or higher self, as your mind is already incapable of supporting itself.

This level is also all about achieving spiritual bliss - one that arrived to you spontaneously. Nirbija samadhi will always be a crucial level in Nirvikalpa as it lets you experience absolute freedom from all your attachments and mental thoughts, especially negative ones.

If you practice contemporary yoga, you will notice Nirbija Samadhi being considered like kundalini activation. It is also possible to define Nirbija Samadhi based on dualism as you can easily perceive it as a non-dual state linked to consciousness. Once you get into this stage after Asmita, you can see yourself finally having the ability to transcend all your illusions of duality. You also get the chance to see through all projection relevant to separation.

With that said, it is safe to say that the experience you will most likely get from this level is that wherein you have a mind, which is formless and radiant. Your mind will finally be liberated completely from conditioning, as well as from attachment and projection. You will be in a stage wherein you enjoy spiritual oneness, which means that your mind has already dissolved entirely.

It is the reason why you can no longer distinguish between object and subject, known and knower, and seer and seen. With the many things you can achieve when you get into this level, it is no longer surprising to see a lot of people describing Nirbija Samadhi as the ultimate state of yoga. Some also consider it as the end product or embodiment of all forms of meditation.

Reaching into this level requires you to get into a deep meditative state – one wherein you let all your intellectual processes and thoughts diminish. Here, you will not see yourself creating karma. It even helps take out the seeds that might plant karma in the future.

With that, you will surely find this level helpful in finally freeing yourself from the somewhat recurring cycle of life and death – one that reincarnates you. With Nirbija Samadhi, you can see your mind merging with Brahman or absolute reality. When that happens, you can finally see this level opening the door for you to reach nirvana.

Sabija Samadhi

There is also what is referred to as Sabija Samadhi, which can be classified as Samadhi with seed. In other words, this specific level has an object of meditation known as pratyaya. One thing to note about Sabija Samadhi is that it covers all Samadhi stages that still have functioning mental inner impressions. Among these stages are Samprajnata and Asamprajnata Samadhi.

Sabija is all about being in a state wherein the actual seeds of rebirth, particularly the five mental afflictions and all traces from your previous experiences, stay active though there is a significant and noticeable reduction in terms of their propensities. Based on Patanjali's yoga sutras, you can see Sabija Samadhi having four primary varieties, with each one being identifiable and distinguishable based on the object of focus. Each of these varieties also represents a progressively subtle variation of your inner existence. These are:

> • Tarka, which refers to the mind revolving around gross objects or particulars
>
> • Vichara, which is all about subtler mental impressions
>
> • Ananda, which is characterized by the mind revolving around the feeling of inner bliss

• Asmita, which comes with mental thoughts revolving only around the "I" sense or the feeling of individuality or uniqueness

Another thing to take note of about Sabija Samadhi is that it has a specific content of mind referred to as Pratyaya, which comes in the form of a feeling, thought, or object. In that case, you can group such thoughts or contents of mind under Samprajnata Samadhi.

You will notice such content on your mind diminishing or disappearing every time you transition to another stage. Each transition helps end all your spiritual strife and reach that specific goal of liberating you from pain and ignorance, giving you the kind of bliss and liberation you are hoping for.

Chapter 7: The Final Stage: Dharma Megha Samadhi

Now we are on the final stage of Samadhi, which is known as Dharma Megha Samadhi. The fact that it is the highest and final stage is proof that it reigns supreme among the various stages and levels related to Samadhi. It is an irreversible state that leads to genuine liberation. Once you get into this stage, you can finally set yourself free from a world filled with dharmas, particularly those that cloud reality.

Setting your Expectations

If your goal is to reach Samadhi, then the final stage that you must aim for is Dharma Megha. Dharma means *virtue*, while Megha can be translated to *the cloud*. One thing you can expect from reaching this stage is that it ends all karma and afflictions. A yogi who gets into this stage is someone who has successfully gained full liberation.

As a yoga practitioner, you can also see yourself being free from all sufferings associated with the external world. The result is Kaivalya, which gives you the chance to experience absolute enlightenment and liberation.

According to Patanjali, anyone can reach this level, even those who have lost their desire to achieve enlightenment or get to know God. The reason is that this final stage of Samadhi is one that you cannot gain by effort. Instead, you can see it revealing itself once you have finally dissolved all your effort. With that, you can people perceiving it as a truly divine gift – one that goes beyond the notions of relative and absolute.

Also referred to as the cloud of virtue, you can expect this stage to bring you liberation and genuine bliss by showering you with pure knowledge and ensuring that you do not get easily tempted by yogic powers that otherwise trigger distractions.

In this state, you get the chance to see without using your eyes, hear without your ears, touch without using your skin, smell without using your nose, and taste without your tongue. This stage of Samadhi is so incredible that even your mere intentions are already enough to create miracles. You just must will it, and you can expect everything to come into being.

Your Journey Towards Dharma Megha: How to Get into this Final Stage of Samadhi

One thing to remember about entering a specific state of Samadhi is that you will most likely experience the thrill of stillness. Once you enjoy this thrill, you will receive a signal that you are close to the specific state you are aiming for (in the case of this chapter, the Dharma Megha).

You will also have a few other distracting experiences that tend to go along with stillness. Some examples of these distractions are extraordinary sensory experiences or clairvoyance. Also referred to as siddhis, these experiences are also identifiable as yogic accomplishments, especially for anyone who never gets to experience Samadhi yet. However, those experienced with Samadhi can view such experiences as obstacles.

Despite that, you must remember that whether the siddhis are meaningless or meaningful for the practitioner or whether they are shallow or profound, their presence is still good. They signify that you are already getting close to the final stage of Samadhi. There is no reason for you to be extremely anxious when you notice these signs with that in mind. You should not also be afraid of them.

Your goal, instead, is to stay focused on your actual destination. Concentrate on reaching your main goal of attaining the ultimate stage of Samadhi, which is Dharma Megha. Also, remember that being anxious, doubtful, and fearful of your journey towards reaching Samadhi may only distract you.

With that said, train yourself not to make a huge deal out of the siddhis you may encounter. Strive to get into the final state naturally. This means applying the principle of most successful yogis, particularly that which involves working hard while still taking everything lightly. You should aim to get to the highest state of Samadhi while still ensuring that you do not make a huge fuss about the entire process.

It is also all about practicing vairagya, an attitude which means non-attachment or dispassion. This attitude is vital if you want to protect and nurture the practice. Also, remember that you need to practice it perfectly to bring yourself closer to the ultimate state. Your goal is to practice yoga in a way that you can get yourself to Samadhi, not just simply conform or adhere to cultural expectations.

In that case, you must stick to the most vital aspect, which is to build a foundation that can support the structure or goal you wish to achieve. Also, remember that the fundamental principles of your fruitful yoga practice that aims to get into the final stage of Samadhi include balance. It is sometimes about attaining balance in various areas of your life, including diet, sleep, thinking, and exercise. Moreover, it is advisable to perform your actions while pairing it with a balanced understanding.

Another thing you must cultivate is a conducive posture. Your posture should be very conducive to your practice. In that case, the best posture would be that wherein you let your trunk, neck, and head form a straight line. It is also essential to relax your shoulders and keep your breath as serene as possible when doing this pose.

Another important thing to do is to keep your breath and mind united. By uniting both their forces, you can focus on just minimal distractions, which is great if you want to concentrate on your chosen object for a longer period. What is even better about prolonged concentration is that it can mature into meditation, which will also mature into the highest level of samadhi.

Your repeated experience of Samadhi, Dhyana and Dharana can help in deepening your memory with the practice. In the succeeding sessions wherein you practice yoga, such memory can push you towards Samadhi while also pulling Samadhi towards you.

Eventually, the entire process will become effortless, which is an indication that you have truly reached Dharma Megha Samadhi, a specific state of Samadhi filled with virtues, particularly those spiritually enlightening and uplifting.

This is where an incredible state of awareness, which is free of desires, such as the desire to get the other benefits offered by Samadhi apart from just attaining this supreme state, arises. It can also be referred to as Nirbija Samadhi, the highest form of Samadhi experienced by Buddha, Patanjali, and other famous sages.

The Three Gunas Resolved in Dharma Megha

When trying to understand yoga's philosophy, remember that all universal matter comes from Prakriti, a fundamental substrate. In Prakriti, the three main Gunas or qualities of energy come out, producing the most vital aspects related to nature, including matter, consciousness, and energy. You must be aware of these Gunas and learn the basics of manipulating them consciously.

With that, you can view it as a powerful and effective method of reducing stress, boosting your inner peace, and bringing yourself closer to enlightenment. It is what Dharma Megha is trying to let you achieve. Getting into this state results in enlightenment and liberation as it frees you from the three main Gunas.

Guna is a Sanskrit word meaning quality, tendency, attribute, or peculiarity. It is an element of reality or tattva in the yoga world, which has a major impact on your energetic, emotional, and psychological states. The three main Gunas that Dharma Megha aims to resolve and remove were developed as vital parts of Sankhya philosophy. However, you will notice that they are presently major concepts in Indian philosophy.

The Gunas are also constantly in flux and tend to interact with each other in a state of playfulness called illusion or Maya. They also have interplay patterns that define the vital qualities of something or someone. Such patterns have a great influence on your life path and progress.

If you are practicing yoga, then being aware of these Gunas can give you a clear guide for making more balanced, harmonious, and peaceful choices, whether you are practicing yoga or you are already out of your mat. You need to cultivate your skill of identifying and understanding the nature of each Guna so you will get to clearly see the oneness' universal truth.

Now, here are the three main Gunas we are talking about:

- **Tamas** - Identified as a state of materiality, inactivity, inertia, and darkness, tamas manifest themselves in the form of ignorance while deluding all beings that come from spiritual truths. Other qualities of this guna are disgust, doubt, helplessness, depression, attachment, laziness, addiction, confusion, apathy, boredom, shame, confusion, dependency, and grief.

- **Rajas** - This state is linked to action, movement, change, and energy. This guna has a nature related to attachment, longing, and attraction. It is the specific guna, which strongly connects you to the fruits of your labor. Other traits or qualities that you can point to rajas are anxiety, euphoria, anger, worry, irritation, chaos, determination, restlessness, rumination, courage, and stress.

- **Sattva** - Resolving this guna can bring you to a state of joy, balance, intelligence, and harmony. It is this specific guna that a lot of yoga practitioners intend to achieve since it minimizes tamas and rajas, thereby increasing your chance of attaining liberation. Other traits that can be attributed to sattva are peace, delight, love, freedom, wellness, happiness, trust, bliss, selflessness, fearlessness, gratitude, satisfaction, calmness, and fulfillment.

Once you get into Dharma Megha and release yourself from the mentioned Gunas or just learn how to manipulate it consciously, you can finally identify yourself with supreme reality, which is known for being beyond all forms of power. This state is also filled with knowledge, purity, and bliss. The good thing about being in Dharma Megha is that it ends all karma and afflictions. As the yogi, expect to be able to get into the ultimate stage known as Kaivalya or full and supreme liberation.

Also, remember that all these three Gunas can build an attachment, thus binding yourself to your ego. By rising above such Gunas originating from your body, you can free yourself from old age, birth, death, and disease, promoting ease in attaining enlightenment. This makes Dharma Megha a truly vital state of Samadhi, especially if you are practicing yoga.

Nirbija Samadhi and Its Link to Dharma Megha Samadhi

Just like what has been indicated in the previous chapter, Nirbija Samadhi is that level devoid of the seed or Pratyahara. It is a non-dual and unconditional state of consciousness, because it has seen through all anticipated and projected situations and conditions. It does not have any conditioning cause since reaching this stage means that all of them were already transcended.

Aside from that, reaching this specific state also means that you have already surrendered all conditional activities. The result is a radiant, empty, and formless mind, which does not contain any generalized and specific projections of anything related to the seer and the seen.

It is crucial to note that the non-dual state presented by Nirbija Samadhi is frequently viewed as the ultimate form of Samadhi. But you also must remember that the fact that non-duality is known for being the opposite of duality means that it is still a function of the latter. If you want to liberate yourself from everything, focus on going over duality until you reach transcendental awareness.

When that happens, you get the chance to experience and transcend the duality of the non-dual state. You can then relate this experience to Dharma Megha Samadhi as such requires the latter's cleansing process. Another thing you should remember about Nirbija Samadhi is that it does not result from accomplished practice.

You can only expect it to occur within the practice when you and the actual practice allow the spontaneous surrender to happen. Nirbija Samadhi is also all about the natural progression that occurs from Sabija Samadhi once your sense of self starts losing power. It frequently happens in life spontaneously, often resulting from the open and direct spaciousness that your mind has cultivated with constant practice.

Upon surrendering each karmic imprint, it is Nirbija Samadhi that will most likely remain. Until such a surrender happens, this state will become just a temporary possibility. After resolving all your karmic imprints, you will notice Dharma Megha Samadhi irrevocably revealing the dualistic nature of the immeasurable consciousness, space, self, and time. It can then create the non-dual embodiment of otherlessness or Kaivalya.

Chapter 8: The Path of Elevation of Awareness

If you want to have an easier time reaching the ultimate state of Samadhi, then you should try to understand the more advanced levels of its different stages and apply them to your daily life. All forms of samadhi can be defined as altered or transformed forms of consciousness. Moreover, all these forms are not part of the experiences of those who are not practicing yoga.

However, note that even real yoga practitioners also notice that different types of samadhi seem to have a huge gap, especially in terms of attainability. This means that several levels set each type or state apart.

Those who do not practice yoga can also obtain a bit of insight on Samadhi and its types and states by spending time reflecting on what makes the experiences between dreaming and waking different. You need to be able to distinguish these two experiences – both of which are major forms of consciousness that everyone can access.

Understanding the Planes of Awareness

Trying to reach Samadhi means getting into a state wherein you can transcend the limits of your mind and your self-identity and body and unite them into something that you can't differentiate. It also requires you to go through the process of meditating using heightened and concentrated awareness.

In that case, you must understand how the planes of awareness work so you can truly get to the kind of consciousness or awareness that Samadhi is supposed to give you. One thing to note about it is that while there are those who get into Samadhi instantly, the more common scenario is progressing through a set of stages or experiences when you try to go your way towards reaching your goal.

The first hint you may encounter is the feeling of genuine peace and joy as well as general well-being. It is possible to attain such an experience through meditation, vigorous exercise, or even by spending time enjoying a moment of solitude with solemn music.

This specific plane of consciousness or awareness can make you experience that state wherein you lose track of time. It causes you to be fully absorbed over the whole experience temporarily. The experience is fleeting, though. Even with that, it can still give a hint on what the future is in store for you as you go through more profound planes of awareness and levels of Samadhi.

Deliberate Samadhi

This is another phase or plane of awareness that you will have to experience when reaching Samadhi. In here, you will notice a steadier level of consciousness. A lot of people also tend to achieve this level through deliberate effort. Reaching this phase gives you the chance to experience yourself being in a specific point of awareness or consciousness existing beyond your emotions, personality, body, and mind.

You are perfectly and fully aware of their existence, though it is also the phase wherein you no longer view them as major components of your identity. Instead, you look at them as if they are tools or instruments you can use eventually. When it comes to personality, you start viewing it as a set of acquired experiences.

Being in this plane or level of awareness gives you the chance to enjoy lasting and profound peace. However, your sense of self-acting as a unique and separate being stays intact.

By reaching deliberate Samadhi, you are also giving yourself the chance to be free of suffering. Keep in mind that it does not necessarily mean not feeling physical pain or experiencing emotions. What happens, instead, is that they serve as actual occurrences within both your body and mind.

Since you already view both your mind and body as tools instead of your real identity, you also get the chance to view suffering as an optional experience. With that, it is safe to say that you bring yourself to a profoundly liberating situation, which can significantly make some changes in your life.

Getting Into More Superior Levels of Samadhi

Being in the higher level of samadhi or superior plane of awareness can make you feel wonderful as it serves as your starting point when trying to experience even further and advanced levels of samadhi. You know that you are already on the higher level if you perceive and see yourself as a significant point of consciousness or awareness existing over your physical self.

Here, you will get the chance to cultivate the skills necessary in exploring other realities and dimensions beyond physical realities. It could be other timelines, manner of being, or lifetimes. During this stage of consciousness, allowing yourself to be in direct contact with what is divine is possible. You can do that through deliberate searching or seeking.

All sages and mystics of spiritual traditions tend to impart the adventures and experiences they have when under these stages. They also tend to impart personal growth, healing and learning they derived from the whole experience.

When you are at this stage, you will have numerous opportunities to explore and serve. Keep in mind, though, that everything here can be categorized as only a phase. You will eventually discover that regardless of how good, ecstatic, and growth-promoting your experiences are, they are still only mainly designed to help you explore duality.

As you go through the process of uniting with the divine, you will most likely strive to progress over the occasional connections and glimpses with it. The goal is for you is to attain the highest level wherein you get to merge with it completely.

But you must also prepare yourself for the challenges you may encounter. The reason is that no matter how varied and incredible your experiences are, there is still a possibility that you retained that sense of your unique and separate self. It could be one that is separate from everything you experienced and from others around you.

It is vital to advance into the highest level of Samadhi, dissolving this unique sense of self that you view as a unique and distinctive being. You may find this stage very challenging but with focus and determination, plus a higher level of awareness; you can get past through it.

Also, remember that while you can't find only a single solution for attaining dissolution, the planes and the process you have followed so far somehow prepared you for this moment. One thing you can do is to relinquish your unique identity as a personality, body, or mind. Doing so can help you in shedding your self-concepts.

You may also want to travel to alternative realities, experience previous lives, and encounter non-physical beings – all of which can instill within you a more expanded sense of your real identity. You may strip away various layers of your identity until everything disappears, or you may want to expend your self-experience in a way that encompasses all things.

Regardless of what you do, your goal when you reach this advanced plane of awareness is to relinquish every sense of uniqueness and separateness and let it dissolve to radiant light and pure bliss that can be merged with the divine.

Divine Samadhi

Of course, the divine Samadhi reigns supreme as this level or state does not have time, place, and effort. Before reaching this specific point, you most likely viewed the universe as a seemingly infinite place full of a limitless number of things.

In divine samadhi, you will not be able to sense anything related to infinity and the universe. You can't experience anything since you are already one with your experiences. Here, you will feel neither unconscious nor conscious. It gives you the chance to be just simply you.

Note that even after you separate your awareness from Divine unity, you can still retain your realized real nature. With that, you can still consciously behave as an individual inside the physical realm. You can do so while retaining your complete awareness of the Divine Samadhi.

Thinking of all the levels of Samadhi and planes of awareness you must go through, you will immediately realize that each one lets you experience growth while on the path of developing your spirituality. You will also discover that every level is extremely beneficial, depending on your specific needs and life circumstances.

Delving Deeper into Consciousness

Samadhi is the ultimate means for you to dive deep through your consciousness after you master the 8-limb yoga as well as the various stages that you need to undergo. Even though Samadhi is the end goal, it is not considered as the end of the yoga practice. As a matter of fact, it is only the start of it. You must keep that in mind if you want to achieve success in this journey.

Here, the ten identified types of samadhi will establish a sequence characterized by awareness or consciousness descending from the superficial to deeper layers and consciousness levels.

It is also crucial to remember that the main objective of practicing yoga is to join. Now the question is, what is it that you must join? The answer is infinite. According to Patanjali's yoga sutras, joining or connecting with infinity is referred to as Kaivalya, which can be translated to isolated or alone. This concept is called absolute infinite by Western minds.

The ten forms or types of Samadhi are sequential phases or stages you need to pass if you want to move from your waking consciousness's relative existence to the actual infinity phase known as Kaivalya. With that said, it is safe to say that yoga serves as the method, protocol, and steps you must abide by to have a direct experience of the infinite.

You need to take steps from relative to the absolute cover of the ten famous types of Samadhi. These ten types include the four that form part of Samprajnata Samadhi, namely Savitarka, Savicara, Ananda, and Asmita, as well as the four composing Asamprajnata Samadhi, namely Nirvitarka, Nirvicara, Ananda to Asmita, and Asmita to Nirbija Samadhi.

The last two types are Nirbija Samadhi and Dharma Megha that will bring you to Kaivalya. It is the time when you reach the feeling of elevation. At this time, you will notice the fullness and totality of awareness and consciousness coming to you. It will also lead to you witnessing your complete consciousness dawning in you and causing your mind to get completely transformed. This results in attaining clarity every time you think. Clarity will also start appearing in your feelings.

It can transform your entire body in the sense that it becomes so alive and full of prana. It eliminates all obstacles from your path, leaving only the memory of lordship and the divine. With that, you can finally dissolve and let go of obstacles and struggles from your mind.

Chapter 9: Kaivalya State

Another ultimate state of Samadhi that you must familiarize yourself with is Kaivalya. It has been touched lightly in the earlier parts of this book, but it is time to give it more attention through this section. Kaivalya is the ultimate objective of Raja yoga. You can translate this term as detachment, isolation, or solitude. It means isolating yourself from Purusha and liberating yourself from rebirth. To attain Kaivalya is always the main reason why you must motivate yourself to attain Samadhi.

Why Should You Attain Samadhi?

There are several great reasons why you should work on attaining Samadhi. The goal should be to attain Kaivalya, your union with the Divine and a sign of complete liberation. However, there are also other incredible reasons why you should try attaining Samadhi – among which are the following:

> • **Increases Your Body's Level of Energy** - One thing that Samadhi can do for you, especially during your meditation sessions, is to raise the energy flow inside your body. It is a vital energy called prana, which forms a major

part of your spiritual body. It has a major and direct impact on your physical body's vitality and energy.

By practicing yoga and meditating to reach Samadhi, you can rejuvenate your mind as it can eliminate all your excess thoughts. With that, you will start feeling more energetic and vibrant. This can also further result in lower stress and anxiety, making it possible for you to sleep better and more peacefully. In that case, you can wake up feeling truly refreshed and more energetic.

• **Improves Emotional Resilience** – Another great reason you must consider attaining Samadhi is to boost your emotional resilience. This capability is extremely helpful during these modern times when controlling emotions is quite challenging.

Keep in mind that just like your physical body, your mind also runs constantly. It chases a wide range of thoughts. It results in an overactive mind, leading to more issues, like poor eating habits, weak immune system, and poor sleep. It is where attaining Samadhi can help.

It increases your self-awareness, making it possible for you to look at yourself at an even deeper level and understand what it is going through. With that, you can boost your emotional resilience, giving you the chance to handle all your afflicting emotions and thoughts, even those buried deep inside your subconscious mind.

Your stronger emotional resilience brought on by Samadhi is also extremely helpful in improving your ability to make decisions. It can make you more emotionally sound, which is great if you want to have an easier time handling tough situations and resolving conflicts.

- **Improves Focus and Mental Clarity** – Another thing that Samadhi can do for you is to improve your mental clarity and focus, which is one great reason to motivate you to attain this supreme state. This state plays a crucial role in building your concentration and focus.

Once you get into Samadhi, you will notice your body's sensations dissolving, giving it complete rest. It can also silence all thoughts that arise in your mind, leaving you with only the realization of being.

By removing all thoughts that have too much weight on your daily life, you will surely feel light after each practice session. You can clear up your mind and notice your load lightening up as your thoughts disappear. This can further lead to experiencing pure bliss.

Aside from the mentioned reasons, you should also try to attain Samadhi because it is the ultimate way for you to connect with the divine. It can improve your spirituality and bring you a lot closer to God. Just make sure that your goal for reaching Samadhi is to attain Kaivalya.

Understanding Kaivalya

As the ultimate reason for attaining Samadhi, it is necessary to learn everything you can about Kaivalya. If you are still unfamiliar with it, note that Kaivalya is the ultimate enlightenment state you can reach. Also referred to as nirvana or moksha, the state of Kaivalya allows you to be completely free and fearless.

Some people have the wrong perception of it, though, as they view it as annihilation or negation. The entire concept revolves around completely isolating your soul from the matter and gaining a complete understanding that genuine happiness has nothing to do with the external world.

Once you attain Kaivalya, you will realize your independence as well as how important it is. If you want to reach this state successfully, then you need to overcome all your attachments and desires. You must release yourself from any alterations and modifications of your mind, too.

According to Patanjali, your soul will only find the end once it realizes enlightenment, freedom, and Kaivalya. However, take note that even if Kaivalya means being in a state of aloneness, you should never confuse it with living in seclusion or loneliness. It is just all about gaining freedom from egoism, aversion, attraction, duality, and bondage.

It also releases you from the cycle of deaths and births. Kaivalya is the final, eternal, and complete union with the pure and real form. Once you are already in this stage, you can refer to yourself as a Kevalin.

How to Attain Kaivalya

Attaining Kaivalya requires you to go through the path of Nirbija Samadhi and Dharma Megha Samadhi. The reason is that these two are considered as the last couple of stages leading you to Kaivalya. This path towards Samadhi starts from Nirbija Samadhi, which is all about having only pure and empty consciousness in existence. It means that what exists is only your self-aware being.

You can get into this state by being at the Asmita level first, which gives you the chance to go to the deepest level of your consciousness. Note that nothing is already left from the Pratyaya upon accomplishing Asamprajnata Samadhi. It can give you a kind of consciousness that can produce a completely different effect, which is the Nirbija Samadhi.

In this stage, you will notice yourself easily overcoming struggles as you adjust to your fully empty self-aware state. You need to face such struggles until you get into the final stage – the Dharma Megha.

One thing to note is that the aphorisms relating to the two stages – Nirbija Samadhi and Dharma Megha – are abstract and obscure. You can see this fact is indicated in the yoga sutras. These aphorisms are also almost not comprehensible. With that said, there is a great chance that Patanjali just wants to relay that when you are in Nirbija Samadhi, you will experience the emptiness between one moment to another.

With that experience, you can train yourself on how to execute Samadhi even if you feel emptiness. If you succeed, then it is safe to say that you have finally mastered and reached Dharma Megha. This will also finally bring you to Kaivalya.

Based on the path of Nirbija and Dharma Megha Samadhi, getting into Kaivalya will most likely cause you to go through different forms of liberation – among which are physical, mental, and spiritual liberation.

Basically, you will be taking a 3-step approach towards finally liberating yourself from everything that might be hampering your path towards Kaivalya, including desires, egoism, attachment, delusion or ignorance, nature, and sinful actions.

Physical Liberation

Physical liberation is most likely the first and most important step you can take as you let yourself a journey towards the path of Kaivalya while taking the routes of Nirbija and Dharma Megha Samadhi. Many consider it the most important step as no one can expect to achieve liberation if they do not release themselves from the chains of their physical body.

This step requires you to set your body free from natural urges, impulses, and limitations. You need to do this release gradually to prevent shocking your body. It is also the time when you must begin controlling specific bodily activities and functions, like thirst, hunger, sexual desire, sleep, breathing, and any desire for physical pleasures.

Aside from that, you need to free yourself and regulate your attachments with your name and your form. One thing to remember about trying to reach Kaivalya is that your fight to be free should start with your body. The reason is that it is the main domain of nature. It is what holds maximum power and strength.

The fact that nature holds a powerful and significant influence on your body makes it hard for even yoga gurus and advanced yoga practitioners to succumb to their natural desires. This is what you have to try to prevent from happening as much as possible. You need to master the art of dealing with all your natural and physical desires and urges, so you will not lose your way and truly push yourself towards Kaivalya.

Mental Liberation

You also need to achieve mental liberation if you want to reach Kaivalya. Remember that your mind is an unstable and restless aspect of your personality. Many also consider it as the most binding and limiting factor for your liberation. The reason is that it is prone to succumbing to external influences and internal weaknesses.

You have to learn how to liberate your mind from the chains of the world if you want to succeed while taking the path from Nirbija Samadhi to Dharma Megha and finally to Kaivalya. It is possible if you control your desires, feelings, concerns, emotions, impulses, and thoughts. You also need to start controlling your attachment, prejudices, greed, pride, egoism, enmity, anxiety and likes, and dislikes.

You will immediately know if you have already achieved mental liberation if you stop being critical, judgmental, angry, fearful, and anxious – among many other negative feelings. In this case, you must do something to cultivate detachment and stay impervious to life difficulties and problems.

Try liberating yourself by preventing external events from bothering you, too. You can implement this approach whenever you practice sameness and equanimity to all pairs of opposites and dualities. Besides that, mental liberation is achievable if you cultivate good virtues and practice detachment, dispassion, compassion, patience, equanimity, tolerance, and forgiveness. Moreover, you need to train yourself to achieve the right and proper thinking, as well as excellent self-absorption, meditation, and concentration.

Spiritual Liberation

Once you finally gain full control of both your body and mind and you purify and fill both with sattva's predominance, you can expect spiritual freedom or liberation to follow naturally. You have to achieve this path if you want Kaivalya to be within your reach finally.

Take note that you can only attain spiritual liberation if you are successful in completely freeing yourself from all forms of attachment, desire, and conditioning. This means that these things should not be around to conquer, disturb, or overwhelm you. Your goal should be to transform yourself into one that is not touched by any impurity or action surrounding you.

In most cases, you can get into this state via detachment, devotion, knowledge, faith, and surrender. Apart from pushing yourself towards getting the best results out of yoga and meditation, you also need to practice liberating yourself spiritually by trying to study the scriptures. Moreover, you must transcend your ignorance, follow scriptural injunctions, cultivate proper discernment, and approach someone knowledgeable about spirituality, like a spiritual master or a yoga guru.

Nothing can also beat your decision to surrender to God and act selflessly and sacrificially devoid of any expectations and desires when it comes to achieving spiritual liberation. The good thing about this state is that everyone can possibly achieve it. You can't test it physically, and attaining this kind of liberation may also be hard at first, but you can still rest assured that it is possible.

Being genuinely free in this sense means you must go through the process of freeing both your body and mind, too. You have to be willing to achieve such kind of freedom. Your goal is to gain full control over both your body and mind, as well as the specific constraints you can subject yourself to. This can result in you living like a free soul, free from any concern or care.

You can also stop yourself from indulging too much in self-perpetuation and self-promotion. You will get the chance to learn and follow the flow of life. By liberating yourself, especially spiritually, you can also open up yourself to various aspects of life without any expectations or fear.

All these are what you will surely be able to experience when you reach Kaivalya. It is the kind of enlightenment that will let you feel genuinely happy with your life, even if you do not have a lot of material possessions.

PART THREE: Samadhi
Applications in Daily Life

Chapter 10: The Benefits of Samadhi Practice

As a yogi, your goal should always be to get into the state of Samadhi. It is an indication that you are successful in your practice. You can consider yourself a true yogi if you went through sufficient practice that makes you master the art of detaching and attaching yourself.

When you get into this state, you can say that you have attained Samadhi, one wherein you also have the chance to gain a full understanding of yourself. In this state, you will connect with the divine and achieve spiritual enlightenment and come to terms with your real personality.

Being the last limb in the yoga sutra, Samadhi completely absorbs your consciousness and allows you to observe better. Most also consider it as the higher meditation level taught in several popular yogic schools.

Another advantage of Samadhi is that the entire process of reaching it gives you the chance to go through stages designed to improve your life's various aspects. With that, it is no longer surprising to see many people applying this practice into their daily lives.

Samadhi Promotes Better Health

One of the known benefits of Samadhi yoga, and the meditations sessions that usually come along with it, is superior and better health. As a matter of fact, various studies, including the ones conducted by the Journal of Psychosomatic Medicine, showed a significant reduction in the number of cases of cancer and cardiovascular diseases among those who meditate and practice Samadhi yoga regularly.

The main reason behind this is that Samadhi meditation provides positive changes in the way your immune system function. The good thing about these positive results and changes is that they last for a long time. The practice even helps in slowing down HIV progression.

Another thing that Samadhi can do for you is to lessen your pain experience as well as brain activation related to pain significantly. It has even been discovered that Samadhi yoga and meditation can lessen more pain compared to morphine and other popular pain relievers.

Among the kinds of pain that this practice can help deal with are migraine headaches, joint inflammation, and lower back pain. Samadhi can also promote better health by lowering the level of stress generated by your mind. Note that stress is a common trigger of some health issues.

It can even lessen the flow of essential energy inside your body, affecting the health of its different parts and organs. By practicing Samadhi through yoga and meditation, you can lower your stress level, which can also lead to better health.

Samadhi Increases your Emotional Quotient

Practicing Samadhi is also good for you as far as your emotional intelligence (EQ) is concerned. Samadhi meditation and yoga practitioners even noticed a significant improvement in the way they handle their emotions after they successfully attained the supreme state.

According to the study performed by the University of Wisconsin, the Samadhi practice helps in boosting emotional intelligence by stimulating activities in various parts of the brain that aid in formulating positive feelings and emotions, like self-control, joy, and happiness. It also reduces activities in certain parts of your brain linked to negative emotions, such as sadness, self-centeredness, and depression.

Apart from that, one can also use Samadhi in calming that specific part of the brain that causes anger and fear. Moreover, it promotes a change in a certain brain section, which has the function of controlling your ability to attain inner peace, especially when you are dealing with extremely disturbing situations.

Yoga and meditation, especially as you relate them to Samadhi, can make you feel calmer and more peaceful and balanced. This benefit is good not only for your physical health but also for your emotional wellbeing and mental health. You will also love the fact that the practice's positive results do not just end after the yoga and meditation session.

Even a short session is already a huge help in calmly going through the entire day and improving your overall health. Samadhi yoga also works in clearing information overload that tends to accumulate daily, thereby contributing to your high-stress level.

It also works in boosting your emotional quotient and intelligence by letting you obtain new perspectives on difficult and stressful situations and cultivate some skills necessary in managing stress. Moreover, regularly practicing Samadhi can boost your self-awareness, lessen your negative emotions, and allow you to focus on the now or present. All these benefits can signify that you will be on your way towards raising your EQ.

Samadhi Improves Brain Functioning

A higher and better brain function can also be linked to the constant practice of Samadhi. Those who constantly do Samadhi yoga, allowing them to meditate along the process, are famous for having better brain activities, specifically in the areas of the brain that process positive emotions.

The practice also seemed to help in lessening activities in certain brain areas linked to depression, anxiety, as well as other unwanted and negative emotions. By meditating, always a part of yoga practice, you can raise the size of the specific brain region linked to positive emotions.

Furthermore, daily meditation works to thicken the specific areas of your cerebral cortex that play a vital role in your memory, focus, attention, and decision-making. Other benefits of Samadhi, as it relates to your brain, are better performance academically, higher IQ, better problem-solving and creative skills, increased memory and focus, and more accurate insights or perceptions.

Aside from that, it is also possible for you to experience better job performance and satisfaction as well as faster reaction time. If you are an athlete or sports enthusiast, you will be glad to know that Samadhi can benefit your brain in ways designed to boost your endurance and energy and improve your athletic and sports performance.

Samadhi Promotes Better Performance in Personal Life and Career

With the amazing benefits that Samadhi yoga provides your mental, emotional and physical health, it is safe to say that it can also play a major role in improving your performance in your personal life and your professional life or career. It can boost your performance at work by improving your productivity.

The main reason is that it frees your mind from stress and makes it more relaxed, resulting in it being able to work more efficiently and effectively. Note that the right part of your brain plays a huge role in crafting new ideas. You can expect this side to work more actively if you do yoga and meditation regularly.

The fact that Samadhi can activate that part of your brain is also the major reason why you can start producing new and creative ideas and designs. Moreover, it can significantly increase your concentration, which can further make you more productive.

Samadhi also has an impact on your personal life. It can make you more mindful, which is good in improving your work relationships and your relationships with other people, like your friends, family, and significant other. This practice increases your mindfulness and lowers your stress levels and risk of suffering from depression and anxiety.

It can even help improve your mood, which is beneficial if you want to communicate well with others and express yourself and your emotions. You will have a much better performance in your personal life as Samadhi yoga also improves your emotional intelligence. This can further result in building relationships easily and naturally.

The fact that Samadhi requires you to meditate regularly also improves your ability to accept others, which is the key to creating a more holistic and welcoming environment at work, at home and in any other places you frequent.

Samadhi Improves Creativity and Focus

Samadhi can also greatly benefit your focus and creativity. It can significantly improve your focus as it teaches you to be present in the now. It is also one of the most widely used and practiced techniques for managing stress. You can expect it to work in that area by reducing your psychological distress and promoting clarity in thoughts.

The constant practice of Samadhi yoga and meditation also contributes a lot to expand the level of your self-awareness. Aside from that, many people always consider yoga a way of life characterized by pure bliss, harmony, balance, and health. You will surely find it useful in tapping into your creativity.

Keep in mind that there is a strong connection between yoga and your brain's creative process. Every time you have creative insights, your brain automatically prepares for it by shutting down all its visual cortex activities. It is as if you are closing your eyes to get rid of distractions, allowing you to focus even better.

Your brain is cutting sensory input and improving the signal-to-noise ratio as a means of retrieving or finding answers from your subconscious. You can liken this act of removing other sensory output to pratyahara, the famous fifth limb of yoga. It is the time when you shut off your mind from all influences coming from your five senses.

With that said, it is safe to say that Samadhi yoga has a strong connection with your creativity and focus. It allows you to be at peace and feel more relaxed, which can stimulate your creativity. The good thing about boosting your creativity is that it also helps hone your problem-solving skills.

Your creative insights will start stimulating your brain, so it can constantly find the best solutions for certain problems. This is beneficial for anyone who wishes to express themselves creatively. Also, in yoga sutras, the remaining three limbs of meditation, complete absorption, and concentration are around to help your mind attain stillness.

One advantage of having a still mind is that it can bring out your intuitive wisdom. With that, you can start living your life with the ability to handle all your daily concerns in a more creative manner.

Aside from that, Samadhi yoga and meditation can also provide you with several psychological and cognitive advantages, like better task concentration, learning, and memory, as well as sustained empathy, introspection, and attention. All these benefits are vital to your creativity.

Other Benefits Offered by Samadhi Practice

Practicing Samadhi yoga can make you feel the meditation session so deeply. It is so deep that you will no longer think about anything else, including the fact that you are doing the practice. With that, the whole process will become more natural for you. Apart from the benefits indicated in this chapter, the Samadhi practice will also let you experience the inner tranquility and peace for which you are hoping. It can boost your emotional stability and improve your ability to control your thoughts.

Moreover, it can make your character pure, establish your intuitive ability and willpower, and boost your vitality and rejuvenation feelings. It can make you feel genuine bliss – the bliss of life as well as that provided by just being yourself.

The practice can also give you an indescribable form of happiness and peace. You cannot describe it in words, but you will be able to feel it wholeheartedly. With Samadhi yoga's ability to establish the feeling of alertness, calmness, and peace, as well as help transform your life for the better, making it a part of you is highly encouraged.

Chapter 11: Training the Body and Mind

Now it is time to learn about a few tips and tricks that will help you train both your body and mind and prepare both, so you can easily implement Samadhi. You need to raise your awareness about the different yoga techniques and forms of meditation guaranteed to make the process of making samadhi a part of your life as smooth and hassle-free as possible.

When choosing the best technique for making Samadhi practice a part of your life, keep in mind that the best one is usually that which can help train both your body and mind. Also, remember that one thing that most yoga practices have in common is meditation. This means that every time you practice Samadhi yoga, you will most likely have to meditate.

To start training your body and mind and prepare it to make Samadhi a part of you, here are the most modern techniques and practical tips known for their effectiveness in changing your life.

Mindful Yoga

One effective technique that you can use to get into Samadhi and ensure that you train your body and mind to accept the practice is mindful yoga. It is a great technique as it mainly focuses on mind and body awareness. It does not solely focus on exact physical posture and alignment details but primarily on raising your awareness about your mind and body.

The concept of mindful yoga is to nurture mindfulness within you with the help of asana as the primary vehicle. It brings mindful awareness to all physical activities, which is a huge help in cultivating a more alert focus on anything you are doing. It can transform such a movement into a kind of meditation. With that said, it is safe to say that mindful yoga is a kind of meditation frequently practiced before a formal seated meditation session.

Another distinctive trait of this form of yoga is that it focuses more on observing instead of reacting. Although observing instead of reacting is a common notion and principle in yoga, this specific practice of mindful yoga is different as it considers the process of observing your feelings and mind extremely important every time you do a pose.

Mindful yoga also requires you to scan your own body while aiming to detect even the subtlest ways of shifting your views on your body, your thoughts and entire sense of self every time you change your pose or stick with it. Also, keep in mind that this technique's main goal is to become more open and curious about everything that you have observed and noticed about your body and mind.

You also need to do it without any attachment or judgment, which is always a key component when trying to reach Samadhi. It is crucial to investigate your bodily sensations completely then release your focus of attention intentionally before changing to the next part you intend to explore.

Make sure to hone your curiosity when practicing mindful yoga. Every time your mind wanders, observe carefully so you can easily detect judgment and irritation as they come, then let your mind go back to your body and breath when it happens. Moreover, you need to devote each practice to at least one of the major foundations of mindfulness. Alternatively, you can work through these foundations sequentially.

Mindfulness of the Body

This foundation is all about raising your awareness about your own body being an actual body. It should constantly remind you that your body consists of several parts, including skin, teeth, bones, lungs, heart, and nails, among many others. Each part is a tiny body found in a bigger entity you call as your body.

By cultivating your own body's mindfulness, you will recognize how impermanent your body is and how it is prone to death, illness, and injury. With that, you must look at it as a body and not the ultimate source of lasting and genuine-happiness.

Mindfulness of the Mind

It is also advisable to devote your mindful yoga practice to mindfulness of the mind every now and then. This foundation does not directly refer to your thinking mind. Instead, it is more about raising your awareness and consciousness. The good thing about devoting to this foundation is that it helps you understand that awareness or consciousness occurs from one moment to another and is based on information that comes to you from various senses and your internal mental states.

Moreover, you will get to understand that your mind can't exist on its own. What appears and exists are specific states of mind based on external or internal stimuli or conditions. By paying attention to how every thought occurs and moves away, you will instantly realize and understand that you will never be your own thoughts. With that, you can learn to avoid attaching your identity to your thoughts and look at your mind exactly as it is.

Mindfulness of Feelings

This specific foundation is all about feelings or emotions, and bodily sensations. Note that it is also possible to subdivide the feelings or emotions just like the mind and body. You can master mindfulness of feelings by understanding that no matter what your present emotion or feeling is – whether it is unpleasant, pleasant, and neutral, you should still be able to observe and completely acknowledge it.

You also must remind yourself that such feelings will dissipate eventually. With the help of this foundation, you will know how to observe feelings whenever they arise, instead of identifying yourself with each one or attaching some forms of judgment to it.

Through mindfulness of feelings, you will realize that feelings are just the way they are, so you should avoid using them to define your true self. By starting to perceive feelings as just natural sensations or emotions, instead of your own feelings, you will come to cultivate them in a way that you can also hone your selflessness.

Mindfulness of Dharma

It is also advisable to cultivate mindfulness of Dharma if you want to reach Samadhi and apply this practice in your daily life. The term Dharma is Sanskrit, which is used in describing natural law or the natural way of things. Also called mindfulness of mental objects, this specific form of mindfulness will let you learn and understand all things around you and make you realize that they exist just as mental items or manifestations of reality.

When cultivating mindfulness of Dharma, it is necessary to practice consciousness and awareness of how everything inter-exists. It also reminds you of the fact that everything is just temporary, so they do not have any self-essence. With that, you can identify yourself more as someone who is more aware of your surroundings and understands what is more important.

Siddha Samadhi Yoga

This technique is a form of yoga that also requires you to meditate. One advantage of Siddha Samadhi yoga is that anyone can practice it with ease regardless of religion, gender, creed, and age. Just make sure that you fully understand its meaning, which is to wake up at that state wherein you accomplished knowledge.

Here are the steps involved in practicing Siddha Samadhi yoga and ensuring that it trains both your body and mind to reach Samadhi and make the most out of it.

- **Step 1** – Be in a comfortable sitting position with your legs crossed. Put each hand on each knee while ensuring that your palms face down. This pose is referred to as drone mudra.

- **Step 2** – With your eyes closed focus on remaining steady. During this stage, expect some thoughts to penetrate your mind. However, during the meditation session, you must try gaining complete control of each thought. Your goal should be to get rid of all your thoughts.

- **Step 3** – Visualize a picture of a yoga guru or saint, then focus on it. Your focus on the visualized picture is a huge help in removing all your unwanted and unnecessary thoughts. You should also visualize or imagine the image being in the middle of both your brows. Concentrate even more deeply and begin visualizing it completely.

- **Step 4** – With eyes closed, chant mantras, or OM loudly. Both the mantras and OM can provide similar effects. Note that when chanting mantras, it is highly likely for you to sense the vibrations around you. One advantage of these vibrations is that they can positively affect your body. The vibrations are what you need to cleanse your body internally and prepare it for Samadhi, which is all about having a divine and supreme feeling.

• **Step 5** - Reaching this step means that you finally obtained full control of your mind, making it possible for you to take charge of it. If that happens, be grateful as it indicates that you are already starting to progress on your spiritual path. Stay in this meditative condition or state for as long as you want.

• **Step 6** - If you are successful in this Siddha Samadhi yoga meditation, you can choose to end this session. Do so in a similar way as when you started it. The end of the session means prompting yourself to come out from the divinity or divine feeling. It is also advisable to let your thoughts penetrate your mind in this step. Your goal is to build awareness and consciousness and ensure that your mind is fully aware of everything surrounding it.

• **Step 7** - Do palming slowly. You can do that by rubbing your palms against each other. Make sure to keep them on your eyes. You may also need to use your palms to cover your eyes completely. After that, you can gradually open your eyes. Let your hands and legs move.

Sahaj Samadhi Meditation

You can also greatly benefit from this form of meditation if you incorporate it into your regular Samadhi yoga practice. This meditation technique comprises Sahaj and Samadhi's words, meaning effortless or natural and a deep meditation state, respectively. With this form of meditation integrated into your Samadhi yoga practices, you get the chance to let yourself indulge in a restful, calm, and deep state of relaxation.

One important thing to remember about Sahaj Samadhi is that the meditation session will be based mainly on mantras. This means you will have to repeat a word or mantra silently and over many times in your mind. Chanting the mantra works to calm down your overactive mind and let you settle into a kind of restful calm that will surely guide you to pure bliss, a promise that Samadhi can fulfill.

This form of meditation also makes it possible for your mind to transcend with ease from being in a turbulent state, which comes from your conscious mind's surface to your subconscious mind's infinite depths, the center of your unlimited happiness and creative intelligence.

Another advantage of this form of meditation is that you can practice it even if you are at home. It is also quick as you can complete it in just fifteen to twenty minutes, enough time to transform your life profoundly. To practice it, be prepared to use some mantras as your anchor. It makes it distinguishable from other methods, like vipassana or insight, that use your breath as the anchor.

Basically, you will be doing this form of meditation by sitting in an easy pose. Close your eyes, then repeat your chosen mantra slowly and repeatedly over your head. Keep in mind that you will most likely notice your mind wandering and thinking of random thoughts during the process.

Do not fret, especially if you are still a beginner. You can just gently and slowly bring back your awareness to chanting your chosen mantra and go on. Once you have mastered the art of stopping random thoughts from coming to you during the session, you can reap the rewards of this form of meditation, including bringing you to the most coveted state of Samadhi.

Other Effective Tips for Performing Samadhi Yoga

Aside from the mentioned techniques, it is also necessary to learn about the basic steps and tips you must go through and follow if you want to have an easier time practicing Samadhi yoga. To get the best results and increase your chance of training both your body and mind for the effective implementation of Samadhi into your daily life, make it a point to follow these tips and tricks:

Prepare Yourself

Before each Samadhi yoga and meditation session, make it a point to prepare yourself for the entire process. You must prepare both your mind and body so you can easily accept the practice. One preparation you must make is to find the perfect spot for the session. Make sure that you look for a relaxing and comfortable spot where you can sit comfortably. Put your hands on both your knees, then close your eyes. This will serve as your starting pose, which is called the mudra.

Master the Art of Controlling Your Thoughts

Note that you can only go down deep into your Samadhi yoga sessions if you stay steady and learn how to control all thoughts running through your mind, especially random ones. Note that various thoughts may visit you during each session, so you must master control and improve your focus, particularly once you start to meditate. Get rid of all unwanted thoughts and make sure that your focus is a hundred percent.

Use Your Imagination

Your imagination can significantly help in improving your focus. One thing you can do is to visualize or imagine an image of your yoga guru. Stay still and try your hardest steadying your mind. Get rid of all fear and anxiety and visualize the image appearing in between your brows. It contributes a lot in boosting the level of your concentration.

Chant Mantras

You can also further improve your focus and concentration on each session by learning some mantras and chanting them. If you do not know even just one, then simply saying "om" would be enough. Avoid chanting it too softly, though. It can produce similar effects as when you express a real chant.

The good thing about including some chants in your sessions is that it can make you feel positive vibrations within yourself. With that, you will most likely get the chance to cleanse your body and have that divine feeling that only the state of Samadhi can offer.

End Each Session with a Newly Gained Sense of Consciousness

Note that the perfect time for you to end each Samadhi yoga session is when you have finally gained the highest level of consciousness. You should be at the stage wherein you have a heightened sense of awareness about the world surrounding you and everything that is within it. With this kind of consciousness, you can start seeing everything in a new light since you are now aware of what truly matters.

Chapter 12: The Unification of Paths

Anyone who intends to reach Samadhi can now access several books and programs with a lot of relevant information that will guide them throughout their journey. With the many yoga resources introduced to the public at present, it is safe to say that you have several paths to reaching Samadhi. But take note that regardless of these numerous paths, you still must go through the three primary stages of Samadhi.

The other programs, techniques, and views about Samadhi yoga are mere modifications of the three stages of Samadhi introduced by Patanjali. You can unite all these techniques, so reaching pure bliss and the ultimate state of consciousness will be a lot easier for you.

Different Types of Samadhi

When it comes to unifying the paths towards your goal of reaching Samadhi, you must learn about its different types. It is the key to understanding Samadhi on a much deeper level. Basically, there are three types of Samadhi that you must be aware of - two of which are among the first couple of stages that you must go through during your journey, namely Savikalpa Samadhi and Nirvikalpa Samadhi. The third type is known as Sahaja Samadhi.

Savikalpa Samadhi

With Savikalpa Samadhi, you can still have thoughts inside a trance. However, such thoughts will not be able to disturb nor perturb the trance. In other words, even if there is a set of ideas and thoughts, you, as the seeker, will still enjoy the divine trance as it will remain unaffected.

Also, note that Savikalpa Samadhi will let you diminish all human awareness and consciousness for a short period of time. It takes around one to two hours and is characterized by the conception of space and time being completely different. With that, expect to feel like you are in a different world. You can unify this type and stage with other methods by understanding that you are just an instrument, and almost everything is already done.

Savikalpa Samadhi can also make you realize that everyone needs to go back to ordinary consciousness. You will most likely encounter various ideas and thoughts coming from different places, but you have an assurance that all these will not have a huge impact on you. Every time you meditate, you stay unperturbed. You will also notice your inner being functioning confidently and dynamically.

However, you should aim to go a notch higher by uniting with or being one with your soul in Nirvikalpa. The reason is when you get united in that specific stage of Samadhi, you will be more adept in eliminating any thought or idea. It will let you get into a trance without the mind – only pure bliss and infinite peace.

Nirvikalpa Samadhi

As what has been mentioned a while ago, you need to push yourself to move on to Nirvikalpa and unite with the soul in this specific stage. Upon entering into Nirvikalpa, expect to feel like your heart is bigger compared to the universe. In ordinary situations, you can perceive the world and the universe as bigger than you are. The main reason is that it is your limited mind that perceives both the world and the universe.

Nirvikalpa samadhi can help you view the universe as just a small dot within your huge heart. With that, you get the chance to experience infinite bliss and make that supreme feeling grow. Nirvikalpa is also the highest form of Samadhi attained by a lot of spiritual masters. If you get yourself into this state, then expect its effects to last for several hours or even days.

After that, you need to come down again. Remember that you will most likely experience certain effects like forgetting your own age and name when you come down. You may also be unable to think or speak properly.

However, the continuous practice of Samadhi, particularly the stage of Nirvikalpa, can help you function normally right after coming down. Also, remember that once you enter Nirvikalpa, you will have that urge to not return to the world. You should avoid that from happening as staying in Nirvikalpa for at least eighteen to twenty-one days may put your soul at risk of not being able to come down again as it will permanently leave your body.

There were several occasions in the past when spiritual masters attained Nirvikalpa and ended up being unable to come down. These spiritual masters were successful in attaining the highest form of samadhi but faced difficulties returning to the world atmosphere and acting like humans again. Note that it would be impossible to operate and work in the world if you are still in the state of Nirvikalpa.

However, it is still possible for divine dispensation to occur. In case the Supreme wants a specific soul to continue working on earth, the Supreme can help find another channel of divine and dynamic consciousness to bring him back to the earth even if twenty-one days have already passed.

Sahaja Samadhi

The highest form of samadhi that you will be able to attain is Sahaja. It allows you to be in the most superior form of consciousness while still working in the physical world. With that, it is possible for you to retain your experience when you were still in Nirvikalpa while doing earthly activities.

Many also consider it as the most versatile Samadhi as it allows you to be a soul while also using your body as the ideal instrument. When you get into this form of Samadhi, you can still do the things that normal and ordinary humans do. The only difference is that divine illumination will supercharge you, especially the innermost parts of your heart.

Being in Sahaja also means that you get united with the master of reality. You can bring yourself at your own will to the highest while still having the ability to come down and bring back your consciousness. Remember that even if you attained the most superior form of realization, reaching Sahaja is very rare.

Only a few spiritual masters got to this state. It is the main reason why the final stage of Samadhi is still the Dharma Megha with the ultimate goal of reaching Kaivalya, instead of Sahaja. Sahaja Samadhi is only attainable by establishing your inseparable oneness with the Highest or the Supreme. Anyone who gets into this state will most likely stay here and will be able to manifest God perfectly and consciously every moment.

Practicing Samadhi and Making the Unification Even More Manageable

Now you have a clear idea about the entire Samadhi practice, its stages, some techniques that can help you practice it, and the basics of unifying every bit of resource associated with it, it is time to leave some parting tips. By just keeping in mind these basic tips, you can practice Samadhi with ease and achieve the unification you are hoping for from all the things you have learned from it.

These tips will surely lead you towards the highest form of Samadhi and restore balance in all aspects of your life.

- **Commit to Practicing Gratefulness** – Make it a habit to spend time each day telling yourself about the things that you truly appreciate and are grateful for. Even if there is only a single thing you can think about, it would still be great for you and the entire Samadhi practice.

- **Master Pranayama or Conscious Breathing** – It is one of those activities that will help you focus on the now. Remember that if you want to achieve success in attaining Samadhi, learning how to be present is the most important. You can do that by focusing on your breath.

  You can start each day centering yourself with your breath for around three to five minutes. Observe your breathing patterns during that short time. Make it a point to breathe calmly and slowly through your nose. Also, concentrate on the sounds produced by your breath and keep your teeth, lips, tongue, and jaw relaxed. Doing this is extremely effective in keeping your mind and body calm and at peace.

- **Master Self-Realization** - Keep in mind that Samadhi is also referred to as self-realization every now and then. Self-realization is all about knowing more about yourself. You have to get to know your true self so you will be able to love and accept who and where you are at the moment. Through self-realization, it would be easier for you to move from a place of truthfulness and honesty. You will also become more accepting not only of yourself but also of others.

- **Meditate** - Make sure that you also continue to educate yourself about yoga, mindfulness, and meditation. Note that based on yoga sutras, the rule is for yoga practitioners to relax their effort's intensity. They can do that by regularly meditating on the limitless energy inside.

You must master the art of meditation as it will also constantly remind you how important it is to slow down. It serves as a reminder that you can't do everything in a single day. With that, it would be easier for you to stay intact and unite with the natural flow of life.

These final, parting tips are simple, but they will surely take you to places if you want to achieve the best results from making Samadhi a part of your daily life.

Conclusion

Samadhi is the ultimate state that anyone who wants to gain the best results from yoga would like to reach. It is all about divinity and the ability to let go of everything that does not matter. Note that you can use any technique you want to reach this state since the most important thing is always the spiritual technology.

Also, you must remind yourself constantly that Samadhi means equality. With that, it is necessary to take equal time nurturing every part and aspect of your being. When trying to implement samadhi into your life, make sure to be willing to do those things that can feed your body, mind, and soul.

Do things that feed your emotions, too. By doing all that, you can surely bring yourself to the ultimate state of consciousness and awareness and make Samadhi a natural part of you.

Part 2: Vastu

The Ultimate Guide to Vastu Shastra and Feng Shui Remedies for Harmonious Living

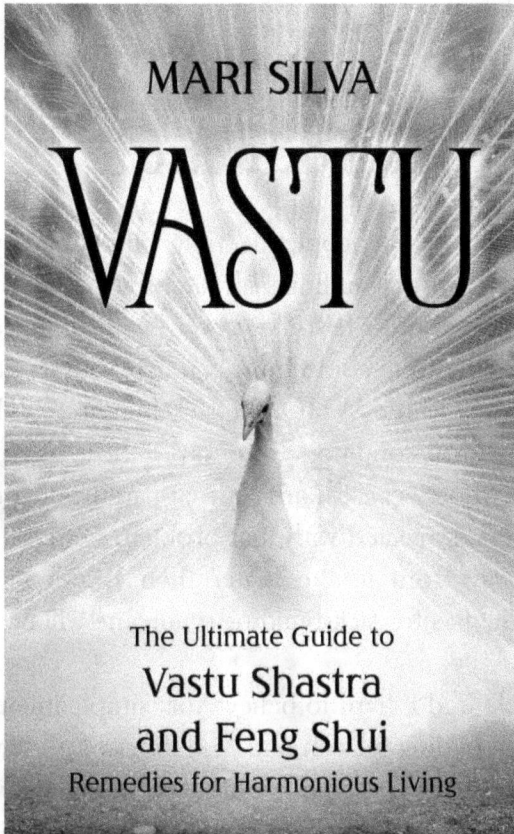

MARI SILVA

VASTU

The Ultimate Guide to
**Vastu Shastra
and Feng Shui**
Remedies for Harmonious Living

Introduction

It's common for many people to view buildings from a purely practical perspective that nullifies all attempts to improve comfort, aesthetic value, or energy. If you've never heard of the 'sick building syndrome,' it's time to become more familiar with its definition and impact. According to the WHO, the sick building syndrome is like an illness or medical condition common to those living in the same building and whose causes are not apparent or obvious. The building is often associated with that problem because the more its tenants are away from it, the better their health becomes. The effects and remedies for sick-building syndrome will be explained in later chapters.

Many people find it hard to believe that simple inconsistencies in room design, building placement, and interior design can cause drastic imbalances in the flow of our lives. However, many correlations and surveys have proven the positive influence of Vastu and Feng Shui designs. Houses and offices built according to the natural laws suggested by these sciences were of great value to our quality of life.

In essence, Vastu Shastra is an ancient Vedic and cosmic science deeply rooted in the theory of the five elements of nature surrounding us. It considers materials, geomagnetic energy, space, wind, and a host of other important natural aspects to analyze the flow of energy going into and leaving our bodies. Vastu Shastra is one of the few ancient architectural sciences that paid a lot of attention to humans' relationship with their buildings. It has established profound connections between a healthy life and a harmonious home or workplace.

Beginners may struggle to dive into a traditional book on a specialized field of science created thousands of years ago. This book is a simple guide that familiarizes you with important concepts and practical applications to use them in your life and line of work. While this book isn't a strictly academic overview of Vastu Shastra or Feng Shui architecture, it blends the different practical uses with contextual backgrounds to offer knowledge to both beginners and people who have dabbled in this science.

The History of Vastu Shastra goes back several centuries, and it's no easy task determining its exact origin due to its ancient nature. The Varahamihira's Brihat Samhita is believed to be the first Indian textual source to hint at a codified science employed to design entire cities and individual buildings. While Feng Shui is often confused with Vastu Shastra with architecture, these two concepts are hundreds, if not thousands, of years apart. It's believed that Feng Shui rooted its practices around the original principles of Vastu. You'll be able to distinguish between Feng Shui and Vastu by the end of this book, as many comparisons are drawn, elaborating further on the core differences and similarities found in both schools of thought.

This book focuses on the latest findings, analytics, and science-driven data related to Vastu and Feng Shui. Even though they have been around for some time, many new concepts are being discovered and recently translated scriptures. It's always best to have an up-to-date view of Vastu if you're planning to put the knowledge to practical use or study it from a closer point of view. The modern approaches to these sciences can differ greatly from how they were originally taught, seeing how the modern world both extends and detracts elements that may not have been in circulation during the sciences' founding.

The concept of living in harmony with nature is no stranger to modern architectural schools of thought and design, but few systems can get in touch with the cosmic frequencies and Vastu can. True harmonious living starts from within and then extends outward to our homes and other buildings we typically spend time in (school, office, library). So, whether you're trying to build yourself a more natural environment or battling the sick building syndrome, this book should guide you through the journey with both ease and expertise.

There is no shortage of books that can provide you with tips on how to enhance your décor or add finishing touches to create a natural home design, but this book is more about utilizing Vastu and Feng Shui to transform mundane buildings into organic and vibrant structures. From design to destructive Vastu remedies, you'll be learning about the true potential of concentrated energy. Finding a balance between a fast-paced modern life and serenely flowing natural energy is not an easy task. It requires an imaginative approach to solving these enduring concerns, which this book will shepherd you through.

Whether you're a DIYer or simply interested in exploring the realms of Vastu and Feng Shui, you'll find step-by-step tutorials complete with detailed explanations of the purpose of the final goal. Planning, designing, building, decorating, and many other processes are considered to allow for a comprehensive read, whose concepts can be applied in almost every building or environment. You'll be able to calibrate the different requirements for each environment with accuracy, thanks to the categorization and independence of each chapter. When it comes to practical uses, you don't need every chapter in this book to achieve your vision since it's designed to work on an on-demand basis.

You'll notice various intersection points between Vastu and Ayurveda, an ancient Hindu medical science. The similarities between them stem from the same foundational concept; the five elements of nature. As you develop more awareness of Vastu's true effects and implications, you'll be able to combine interior design, architecture, food, herbs, and aromas into a balanced ecosystem that ensures your body is at its most optimal state of health.

Chapter 1: A Brief History of Vastu Shastra

Vastu Shastra, the most famous Indian architectural paradigm, is known for having considerable benefits in terms of balance, harmony, and prosperity. Since most westerners aren't familiar with this ancient art, many believe it holds no real merits. However, this could not be further from the truth. Vastu Shastra has carved a place for itself as one of the most influential holistic sciences. Because learning more about this art is the only way to dispel the myths that surround it, this chapter focuses on the origin of Vastu Shastra and the misconceptions it's commonly associated with.

What Is Vastu Shastra?

Perhaps the easiest way to understand Vastu Shastra is to translate the term into English. Briefly, the word "Vastu" means "architecture," while "Shastra" means "science." Vastu Shastra is the "science of architecture." This science is employed as a guide for construction to guarantee harmony with the five elements of nature, also known as "Pancha Bhoota." These elements make up earth, fire, space, air, and water. At its core, Vastu Shastra is the science of directions and placements, and it stems from the belief that placing these elements in any setting can directly affect the flow of energy in the space. Since this art was first established seven thousand years ago, it's fair to say it has had time to develop and become easier to understand. As opposed to its early days, Vastu Shastra isn't as hard to comprehend now or considered knowledge that only engineers and architectures can leverage. On the contrary, even the average person can use the principle of Vastu Shastra to increase their wealth, spiritual and financial, and live harmoniously with nature. To understand how Vastu Shastra links directions to natural elements, here is a breakdown of where every element should exist for ultimate prosperity:

Earth: With the principles of Vastu Shastra, earth is considered the most important natural element. Because earth surrounds us, it doesn't have an optimum direction. Now, for those looking to buy agricultural lands, the ultimate placement should be southwest, as this direction governs longevity, which helps the land stay in good shape and produces bountiful harvests for longer.

Water: Water comes in many forms, including ponds, rivers, oceans, and even rain. Northeast is closely related to prosperity and wealth, so, according to The Vastu principles, water should be a northeast element. Vastu Shastra's experts believe this placement to be highly auspicious.

Fire: Southeast governs food, cooking, and fire. Since fire is a southeast element, experts recommend that homeowners place their kitchens in this orientation.

Air: Northwest is closely associated with enmity. As per Vastu Shastra's rules, placing windows and doors in the northwest direction is a surefire way to release negative energy and keep a place properly ventilated.

Space: Space is the element that maintains the balance of any setting. To ensure that the energy in a specific place remains balanced, be it a house or an office, plenty of open space should be left at its center.

Who Should You Invest Time in Learning the Principles of Vastu?

As we've mentioned, Vastu Shastra is all about living in harmony with nature, which is why it's an art that all people can benefit from regardless of their education or financial situation. But those who are tired of stumbling over hurdles and feel like their life is not going the way it should, can make great use of Vastu, as the lack of harmony they feel might result from not being in sync with nature. Furthermore, people who are on the market for a house may also benefit from Vastu Shastra since it can help them make sure the proper flow of energy in their new home. It's worth mentioning that the effect of Vastu Shastra can be felt either instantaneously or after a while. So, you must be patient to reap the results you want.

The History of Vastu Shastra

Vastu has been a significant aspect of Indian culture for thousands of years. Perhaps the earliest mention of such art was found in the treatise called "Mayamatam," which was written by the architect Maya—an influential figure in ancient India. The treatise was later discovered in 1934, becoming the first inkling of Vastu Shastra in antiquity. The excavations in Harappa, which aimed to unveil the Indus Valley Civilization, also found traces that hinted Vastu Shastra's principles in creating buildings and sewers. Interestingly enough, this elaborate architectural planning only was widely employed in other countries in the nineteenth century. Moreover, Vastu Shastra is mentioned in Indian poetry, particularly in the two Sanskrit epics "Mahabharata" and "Ramayana", which explore popular ancient Indian tales. Since this science was first used to build temples in ancient India, there are many mentions of it in sacred Hindu texts, such as Garuda Purana, Vishnu Purana, Matsya Purana, Agni Purana, and Skandha Purana.

The Story of Vastu Purusha

The story of Vastu Purusha explains the origin of science's principles. Generally, there are two versions of this story. Here is a rundown of each version:

Version 1

Shiva, the third god of the triumvirate and the lord of destruction, was engaged in an arduous fight with a demon. Due to the sheer strength of the demon, Shiva was growing tired and sweated. The drops of sweat that fell from his forehead birthed a creature called Vastu Purusha. Because he was born out of struggle, the creature was immensely hungry and had an appetite for destruction. His rampage struck fear into the other deities' hearts who thought he would devour the whole universe. The creature was too strong to contain on their own, though. So, they sought Lord Brahma, the god of creation, to find a solution to that conundrum. Brahma pushed Vastu Purusha, making him fall, after which he and the other 45 gods prevented Vastu Purusha from standing up by sitting on him. Knowing he was defeated, Vastu Purusha begged for mercy, claiming that none of it was his fault, that he was created this way. Because Brahma was a merciful god, he let him live and helped him satiate his hunger by allowing him to receive offerings from the people living in the houses built on him. In return, he promised to offer them prosperity and guard their health. Although, if they didn't satiate Vastu Purusha, they would face the consequences of his wrath.

Version 2

Lord Brahma was experimenting with his powers, attempting to bring new creatures to life. He created a gigantic man with an insatiable appetite. Brahma didn't give the man a name, and he let him satisfy his hunger as he saw fit. The man grew in power and body to the extent that he cast a shadow on Earth. As his powers grew more destructive, Lord Shiva and Lord Vishnu, the preservers of creation, asked Lord Brahma to stop the carnage the man was causing. As he realized his mistake, Brahma rushed to request the aid of Astha Dikapalakas, the gods of the eight directions, to help him take down the man. Other gods also joined in the fight, and they all pinned the man facedown. The man cried and begged for mercy. Lord Brahma was not known to kill any of his creations, which was why he gave the man the name "Vastu Purusha" and asked him to guard the families' prosperity that built structures on him in exchange for taking gifts from them to ward off his insatiable hunger. Just like the first version of the story, Brahma allowed Vastu Purusha to punish those who failed to extend offerings.

As you can deduce, both stories focus on keeping Vastu Purusha satisfied by implementing the guidelines of Vastu Shastra. Harmony and prosperity are always the results of following these rules. But disregarding them means angering Vastu Purusha and facing adversity.

Myths About Vastu Shastra

Vastu Shastra and Feng Shui; Two Sides of the Same Coin

Since both concepts focus on the art of placement, some people confuse the Indian science of Vastu Shastra with Feng Shui. Feng Shui not only originated in China, but it's also a lot younger than Vastu Shastra. While Feng Shui draws on the principles of Vastu Shastra, it disregards some of Vastu's natural elements, such as space and earth. Vastu Shastra places more emphasis on concepts like weight distribution.

Vastu Shastra Is Superstition

Many propagate the belief that Vastu Shastra is merely a superstition built to trick people into thinking that their lives can change drastically by implementing its guidelines. This is just a misconception. Vastu Shastra is real science; it's built on astronomical and architectural knowledge. There's a spiritual dimension that goes into Vastu Shastra, but it isn't an integral part of it. It goes without saying that this science's principles aren't a magical remedy to all your problems, but following them can still have a positive impact on your life.

You Must Use Indian Furniture to Properly Implement the Rules of Vastu Shastra

Even though Vastu Shastra is an Indian art and practice, you mustn't limit yourself to Indian furniture when designing your space. Vastu Shastra is simply the science of placement, so it is where you put your furniture, not where it comes from, or what it looks like. If you are a fan of the rustic chic, bohemian, or even gothic aesthetic, choose the pieces that strike your fancy. Just be careful to follow Vastu's Shastra's rules of placement.

Feng Shui and Vastu Shastra Can Be Used in Tandem

Because Feng Shui and Vastu Shastra are both placement systems, there are people who think that using them together is the best course of action. However, this can do more harm than good. While the two systems might share several similarities, some of their rules contradict each other. So, it'd be wise to stick to just one system instead of blending two design paradigms fundamentally different.

The Principles of Building Vastu Temples

Most Indian temples are built according to the guidelines of Vastu Shastra, but before we give you examples of these sacred places, you need to know some of Vastu Shastra's rules for building temples. These go:

Shrines and entrances must face the East since it's the direction in which the sun rises. This gives it holy prominence.

Temples can have up to four entrances, with two in the east and the remaining ones facing north. But if the temple has only one entrance, the first rule applies.

The plot of land the temple will be built on should always be square-shaped or rectangular because circular, triangular, oval, or any other irregular shape is inauspicious. These shapes encourage the flow of negative energy and are considered unfavorable.

Water fountains should be placed in the east or northeast because these directions are closely related to wealth and prosperity.

If the temple has a kitchen, it must be in the southeast because this is the fire element's direction.

Temples Built According to Vastu Shastra's Principles

As you now know, most Indian temples follow the rules of Vastu Shastra, but perhaps the most famous one is Tirupati Balaji Temple. This engineering marvel was built in 300 AD as a testament to the outstanding legacy of Vastu Shastra. With over 40 million yearly visitors, Tirupati Balaji Temple remains one of the most praiseworthy creations of Vastu Shastra. Its foundations are still as strong as they were almost 1700 years ago!

In the Himalayas, Kedarnath Temple is another product of Vastu Shastra. Destructive floods left the towns near the temple in ruins. Surprisingly, though, Kedarnath Temple was not affected one bit. This proves that the principles of Vastu Shastra are the key to establishing long-lasting buildings that can stand tall in the face of natural disasters.

Vastu Shastra is a brilliant system and philosophy to investigate to achieve harmony in your life. Given its long history, it's a tried-and-true method of ushering in prosperity and wealth. Now that you know more about it, it's time to implement its guidelines to organize your house and workplace. Keep reading to learn more about these unique principles.

Chapter 2: Basic Feng Shui Principles

Feng Shui is an ancient Chinese philosophy that brings balance and harmony between elements. You may have preconceived ideas about Feng Shui, like how you can optimize the elements in your western décor. But that's only the half of it, as it can also bring positive energy, balance and promote energy flow to your physical and mental health. Because we're only familiar with furniture placement in terms of interior decoration, the thought of deriving energy from spatial arrangements can strike as a novelty. In the following chapter, we will explore this phenomenon and discover how you can implement Feng-Shui to leverage this energy in your home or workspace.

What Is the Chi?

Before we delve into the details of Feng Shui, there are basic concepts we need to understand first, such as Chi. In the practice of Feng Shui, Chi is the universal energy that permeates everything around us. It exists everywhere, both inside and outside man-made structures. Chi energy can have different forms, like Prana, Life Force, Ki, or Qi. Since it's a spiritual energy that can be channeled through different vessels, Chi can have multiple expressions that range between the positive and the negative. As for your body, Chi energy can move through three *dan tiens*, or three gateways: the heart region, the pelvic area, and the third eye center. You may have touched on this subject in your yoga class, as Chi is often employed in spiritual exercises.

The word Chi is of a Chinese origin, while Ki is Japanese, and Prana is Indian. Because this energy is purely spiritual, it is controlled via intangible channels and is harnessed through your body. Chi energy lies far from what we understand about the scientific energy and how it's harnessed. Chi energy cannot be converted into physical energy that can be used and measured in concrete, scientific terms. It can only be felt as you focus on your body, something which you can achieve through spiritual exercises, such as yoga or meditation.

Different Expressions of the Chi Energy

One of the most common expressions of the Chi energy is found in Yin and Yang characteristics. It can exist in two contrasting energies with the same origin. Another one of its manifestations can be sensed in the energy circulating throughout your body. This energy can be channeled to specific organs or limbs if you divert your mental faculties to that area. In doing so, this body part's temperature will rise, which proves the truthfulness of the Chinese saying, "Chi follows Yi," as Yi is your attention or focus. You can also find various expressions of the Chi energy in martial arts, yoga, orgone therapy, reflexology, pranayama, and chi kung. Because these practices were developed to enhance their users' mental and spiritual faculties, Chi energy will always be present in such activities.

What is Feng Shui?

Now that you know that the Chi is an integral part of the Feng Shui, you can better understand how to leverage it. Feng Shui mainly focuses on implementing harmony in one's environment. This harmony will channel out the Chi energy to the area surrounding this environment, which will affect people within the vicinity. Feng Shui can bring positive changes to the environment once the placements and adjustments are made correctly. It will influence space, landscape, and time. Harmony between elements brings balance, much like the balance between the Yin and the Yang. Feng Shui also aims to instill a sense of balance between man and nature and between Chi and the five elements. In Mandarin, Feng means 'wind,' while Shui means 'water.'

The Three Basic Concepts of Feng Shui

1. Yin and Yang

The concept of Yin and Yang is relatively straightforward. As you may already know, it implies continuous change, harmony, and a connection between two contrasting elements. It creates balance and acknowledges it as an essential and formative process of nature. The Yin-Yang symbol is central in Chinese philosophy and has been an important part of the Chinese culture for centuries. An example of the Yin and Yang energy is inner and outer energy, light and darkness, and movement and stillness. A combination of two contrasting elements will create harmony and stability, creating an equilibrium. This balance can be tampered with once one element overpowers the other.

2. Qi

While people interpret the Qi as another expression of the Chi energy, others believe it to be another spiritual force that is the product of abstract and real elements, like sunlight, color vibrations, air movement, water flow, our thoughts and feelings, etc. Invariably, this energy will affect how we feel in a certain place according to how harmony and balance are incorporated.

3. The Five Elements

In the eyes of a Feng Shui practitioner, the world comprises five elements, all of which must be in harmony to make a room feel proportionate, peaceful, and spiritually soothing. If these elements are not balanced well, the room won't harbor a positive and energizing appeal. It is important to take these five elements into consideration the next time you arrange your room or any habitable space:

Wood: It symbolizes creativity, strength, flexibility, intuition, and strength. Too much wood will evoke stubbornness and rigidity, while too little of the element can create stagnancy and depression.

Earth: This element generates feelings of balance and stability. An earth-balanced space can make you feel grounded, secure. If that element is overabundant, it will evoke heaviness or seriousness. Too little of that element will instill disorder and chaos.

Fire: Unlike the two previously listed elements, the fire element will spark enthusiasm and may even improve leadership skills. It is a symbol of boldness, inspiration, and creativity. Too much of that element can increase impulsiveness or aggressiveness, whereas too little can make you lack creativity and experience coldness and low self-esteem.

Water: Wisdom, emotions, and insightfulness come from this element alone, which is why it must be balanced in any environment in which it is placed. When water exists in great quantities in an area, it can make you feel socially overwhelmed. In contrast, too little of that element will evoke feelings of loneliness, isolation, and apathy.

Metal: Logic and clear thinking are typically associated with this element. If there's too much metal in a room, it will make you overly critical and reckless, while too little of this element will hinder your critical thinking abilities.

Through these five elements, you can achieve Yin-Yang balance and channel Qi energy properly through space. This is why you must balance out each element delicately. For example, the wood must be placed in vertical shapes so it can mimic the appearance of tree trunks. The wood shade should vary between browns, greens, and blues to resemble the colors of leaves, the sky, and flowers. You can also use house plants and miniature trees in your areas, such as the Lucky Bamboo or peonies, to achieve this. Wood furniture, fresh flowers, and natural fabrics will help you strike this equilibrium just as well.

The Earth element will make you feel grounded and promote a sense of stability. To achieve balance in this element, you must use decoration items in earthly tones, like blue, green, yellow, red, and brown. You may also use images of natural landscapes, such as beaches, forests, or mountains, and hang them on your walls. A room with a low profile kept to the ground will also help you achieve this balance.

Fire is very dynamic, so you must be careful with that element's placement to strike an ideal balance. Many homeowners simply exploit natural sunlight and use candles, but you can improve that balance with incandescent light bulbs and electronic equipment. Decorative pieces in red and golden shades can also be great assets to accomplish a fire harmony.

To incorporate the water element into any space, you'll want to add dark, deep, and glossy tones. You can use reflective surfaces as well by adding mirrors, but you may also integrate gazing balls or any other reflective surfaces for that purpose l. Wavy or asymmetrical shapes will help create water balance. If you're a fan of fish tanks, fountains, or water features, you can use them to create that balance.

Metal balance can be easily achieved through various elements. For example, you can use anything made of metals, like aluminum, iron, silver, copper, or bronze. You may also scatter around rocks or stones if you have decorative pieces made of these materials.

Neutral and pastel colors can be effective, so integrate them into the room's color scheme.

The Bagua Map

Feng Shui practitioners use Bagua maps for décor plans. It's ideal for analyzing energy in any given space and giving you useful pointers on which elements require more emphasis to strike an elemental balance. The Bagua map comprises nine quadrants, which include elements and colors associated with these elements. These quadrants typically pertain to wisdom, career, love, fame, wealth, health, and people. If you don't know how to use a Bagua map, you can simply lay it over your floor plan such that it displays the nine quadrants and the alignments of the room. These maps are often used on floor plans, but you can just as well use them in smaller spaces.

Vastu Shastra vs. Feng Shui

Similarities

As established, Vastu means 'architecture' or 'dwelling,' and Shastra means 'science,' whereas Feng means 'air' and Shui means 'water.' Nevertheless, the differences between these two concepts extend way beyond semantics. Both have a common origin and are based on the belief and study of cosmic energies. Their philosophers believe that permeating energy (Chi and Prana, respectively) controls the flow of energy through spaces and even the human body. Both concepts posit that the center of any house is a powerful pool of energy where the force of all elements combine and intertwine. Vastu Shastra and Feng Shui suggest their own remedies to fix energy imbalances in any space.

Differences

As mentioned earlier, Feng Shui is rooted in the belief of existing spiritual energies, while Vastu presents a scientific basis to it. Feng Shui also focuses on geographical considerations for optimal effectiveness. It also works on creating a more conducive way of life by increasing the amount of positive energy in your home. In contrast, Vastu Shastra's theory dictates rules for building homes, as evidenced by the guidelines for constructing temples, which were laid out in the previous chapter. Color schemes for a house according to the presets Feng Shui are soothing pastel colors like cream, white, and beige, while color patterns of the Vastu Shastra guides range between bright colors, such as red and yellow. Moreover, the south is considered the most auspicious direction for Feng Shui, while the Vastu Shastra holds that the north is the best orientation and is a source of magnetic energy.

Chi and Prana

People believe these two energies are the same, much like God in Abrahamic religions. While this belief might have some truth to it, there are still subtle differences between them. Chi is a life force that finds its origins in early traditional Chinese medicine. It moves through the dan tiens, which work like the chakras, but they differ because they only pass through three gateways: the pelvic area, the heart region, and the third eye center. Prana works similarly to the Chi, but it comes from ancient India's Ayurvedic and yoga traditions. It also moves through pathways called the nadis and is commonly associated with the seven chakras.

You can now see that both the Vastu Shastra and Feng Shui present comparable qualities, as they both operate in similar ways and similar harness energies. However, it is up to you to explore both of their fascinating theories, parse through ancient philosophies, and follow either of these traditions. Once you delve deeper, you can decide which one resonates with you the most and integrate it into your home and lifestyle.

Chapter 3: Harmonious Living: The Modern Perspective

Our houses are our safe havens. The outside world is fast-paced, loud, stressful, and crowded. The only place we must relax, and recharge is our homes. Since we've strayed away from taking good care of our living spaces, the percentage of people affected by sick building syndrome (SBS) is on the rise. Paying attention to your home's design while factoring in balance, color, and harmony is primordial. This comes naturally to many people. However, what most homeowners fail to achieve is a proper spiritual balance in their homes. Harmony and unity are perhaps the most important aspects that anyone who is interested in the interior design must know. To re-invite harmony into our homes, it's important to step back and get back to basics. For this, we need to identify and understand the problem at its root.

What is Sick Building Syndrome?

This syndrome is largely prevalent in people who've just moved into a new place. Have you ever changed homes only to notice that you're constantly getting sick? You might catch the flu back to back or suffer from chronic exhaustion. Recurring symptoms of illness or general feelings of unease that keep getting worse with time are obvious signs you are experiencing SBS. Typically, the severity of the symptoms increases the more time you spend in the building. People may even notice an immediate relief once they step out of their new living environment, albeit temporarily. It's also worth mentioning that the syndrome isn't just limited to houses; SBS can manifest itself in corporate offices, apartments, and all sorts of buildings or structures. However, when the syndrome is linked to the place where you should be relaxing and resting, this can become highly detrimental to your physical, mental, and emotional health. In-office settings, SBS might cause a marked lack of productivity, an inability to focus, physical issues, and an overall disrupted work performance. This condition is commonplace in buildings where occupants begin noticing minor symptoms and signs until they get worse and face great setbacks in their professional and personal lives. It's been estimated that nearly 30% of new, renovated, or remodeled buildings, residential or commercial, can engender this issue for occupants.

Sick Building Syndrome Symptoms

It's no secret that we spend most of our days indoors nowadays, be it the office, university, school, home, or else. This means that our likelihood to develop SBS is now higher than ever. Sick building syndrome can be identified when a group of people (neighbors, coworkers) shares the same symptoms, with a frequency more than what is normal, and without an obvious explanation for their uneasiness. Usually, the symptoms' acuteness varies from person to person and according to the duration spent in the building. Among many, the most common symptoms include red, tired, or watery eyes; irritated, runny, or congested nose; difficulties in swallowing with irritation in the upper airway, a sore throat, and frequent rash and skin irritations. Other symptoms that can hinder your productivity and wellbeing are lethargy, migraines, irritability, along with diminishing concentration, and a shorter attention span. These symptoms do not impact a person's performance at work, the state of their relationship, and their sociability. They also take a significant toll on their overall quality of life, both inside and outside the home. The real problem happens when the building in question is a daycare center or a medical facility, where occupants are likely to be more vulnerable. This syndrome can also negatively affect the dynamics of workplace environments, translating into increased absenteeism, staff turnover, and crippled performance. While closing or demolishing offices due to SBS is rare, its consequences almost always lead to higher operating costs and loss of profit. The repercussions can be frightening. Reversing these symptoms is doable once you learn how to bring harmony and unity into any space.

Buildings and Climate Change

As much as we hate to admit it, our fast-paced, digital-dependent, consumer-based world is likely to toll the bells of civilization as we know it. Fortunately, a growing number of people are becoming conscious of their actions and the consequences they hold. Over the past couple of years, many have realized the true extent of our reckless, consumerist behaviors and their effects on the planet. More than ever, the only way to curb the global issue of climate change is by reducing our amounts of CO_2 emissions. While climate change and global warming are often used interchangeably, there's a key difference between the two terms. The former refers to the long-term increase in Earth's temperature caused by harmful man-induced activities, whereas the latter is a more general term that denotes the warming effect caused by both the planet's natural cycle and human activities. This endemic problem intensified in scope starting in the 1950s, at a time of post-war reconstruction and global industrial production. While the Earth's temperature used to increase only by 1-degree Celsius per decade, this has jumped to 1.2

degrees Celsius per decade ever since. Before 2020, it further increased to hit the 2.0-degree Celsius mark right by the outbreak of the COVID-19 pandemic. Through science and statistics, we've realize that humanity had to endure a sanitary catastrophe, which brought about paralysis and stagnation all over the world. This signals we collectively need to step back and get perspective on our planet's state. Restoring our bond with nature appears as the only viable way to curtail a potential global catastrophe.

Upon looking closely at the biggest pollution sources in our day-to-day lives, the damage is mostly taking place in our buildings and homes (aside from industrial production, global trade, transportation, etc.). A major part of addressing this problem is to analyze our own habits and patterns. This doesn't simply concern what we do in our houses and buildings, but it's also a matter of how our buildings are designed, constructed, the way we use them, along with the locations and types of terrain we choose.

Carbon Footprint

Two important variables must be factored in to reach an estimate of our buildings' carbon footprints. The first one pertains to the amount of energy that's generated and required for constructing and operating buildings. This accounts for roughly 36% of global energy use. The second aspect is the resulting emissions from daily activities, estimated at around 39% annually. Evidently, these figures should not be taken lightly.

Now, to understand the root of the problem, we need to consider two important parts that go into the equation. On the one hand, there's the day-to-day use of energy, which can also be called "operational carbon footprint." On the other hand, we find all the energy expenditure related to the manufacturing of building materials, the transportation of these materials to construction sites, the actual construction process, with all that it entails (electricity and gas use, machinery, labor, etc.). While the operational carbon footprint is virtually impossible to alter, the second aspect can be put under control by minding our actions and allocating resources properly. The carbon footprint of buildings that results purely from construction operations is expected to diminish by nearly 30% in the year 2030, all thanks to the Paris Climate Agreement that aims to limit the rise of global temperature rate only to 1.5 degrees Celsius.

What Can We Do?

Now that we have a better grasp of these contemporary challenges, we should take concrete action to put a stop to all the harmful practices we've engaged in for decades, intentionally or otherwise. A popular, deep-rooted belief states that reducing carbon and greenhouse emissions can only happen once we learn to exploit and control nature in newer ways. This couldn't be further from the truth. Such a conceited and human-centric approach ignores the fact that humanity is only a lost dust speck in the vastness of the universe and that the forces of the universe rule us, not the other way around. Nature simply cannot be tamed. Instead, we must bring harmony back into our lives and learn how to be in sync with our environment. Immersing ourselves in the beauty that nature holds will teach us how to deal more with our surroundings in smarter, more reasonable ways, rather than exploit them for luxury or profit. Ultimately, incremental changes and subtle lifestyle adjustments (energy saving, recycling, use of eco-friendly materials) can make a world of difference and help sustain the planet for decades to come.

Harmonious Living and Unity

While many people will confuse harmony" and "unity," but in truth, there is a major difference between these two concepts. On the one hand, you may think of unity as a design philosophy that seeks to establish patterns by using the same shapes, colors, and materials to put together coherent and balanced spaces. But harmony is the feeling of spirituality and 'sense' that you get from your house's design. This is when Vastu and other ancient paradigms prove their worth and relevance in the modern world. Nowadays, we need a touch of harmony and unity to turn our houses into homes that combine practicality, aesthetics, and relaxation while enabling us to connect with our surroundings.

Several people wonder why the look and feel of their homes are so bland and lifeless, despite having paid a fortune to perfect it and design it to their image. Seven essential principles help bring any interior design together; all must be in perfect balance with one another. Here is a brief run-through of each one:

Theme: Absent a unified theme throughout the house, you will feel chaos seeping in without understanding the real reason. A strong theme is the foundation of your design, in which every shape, material, and color work toward fulfilling.

Rhythm: Every house's rhythm manifests itself in repeated colors, patterns, as well as matching shapes and sizes. While maintaining the rhythm throughout the house is essential, some interruptions with focal points and colorful highlights can add depth and value to your design vision.

Repetition: When a certain element is recurrent throughout different areas of the house. Too little or too much repetition can affect your space in negative ways. The key is to focus on a singular feature of the house (a color, a piece of furniture, a décor item) which you like and place it in different rooms, but in moderation.

Continuation: In a similar vein, this element is achieved through the extension of a certain pattern or line in more than one area to bring these spaces together with a united sense. It can be the color of the walls, a wallpaper design, or the type of flooring. Integrating continuity is the best way to incorporate unity while retaining the uniqueness of any home.

Similarity: The major difference between similarity and repetition is that, with repetition, you are copying the same pattern, color, or shape again to reuse it in another area. In contrast, the similarity is the use of a specific design that seems repeated but shows a characteristic that makes it unique every time (notably geometric patterns). When perfecting this element, your house will radiate unity and balance.

Perspective: Finally, the element of perspective entails creating depth through different dispositions and arrangements, which makes a home's features stand out yet retain their unity.

Harmony and unity are two ancient concepts that still bear a lot of relevance, especially given everything the world is enduring. After understanding the fundamentals of these two concepts and how essential they are, we can delve deeper into Vastu's concepts and applications for harmonious and comfortable living.

Chapter 4: Vastu Shastra Essentials

In the previous chapters, we introduced you to the history of Vastu Shastra and how it remains relevant in today's world, along with the importance of harmonious living. In this chapter, we will walk you through the essential principles of Vastu Shastra and how each precept impacts the overall balance of energies in any space. As you'll come to learn, the different elements of Vastu complement each other to form a workable framework that you can apply to reap its benefits in all aspects of your life, from the home to the workplace. Without further ado, let's dig in!

The Importance of Energy Balance

Years ago, Albert Einstein concluded that everything we know and experience is pure energy. Everything around us, from objects to emotions and sounds, is all made up of energy. Even us humans, our physical and spiritual existence is an embodiment of an intricately balanced, energetic field. When this balance is disrupted, this is when we suffer, physically, mentally, and emotionally. This all brings us to the Vastu teachings and how their purpose is to utilize various features, such as colors and the directions of objects in any space, to restore the energetic balance of its occupants. With that in mind, we'll move forward to expand on the tools of Vastu Shastra and how they can effectively promote this harmonious balance of energies.

Despite being an ancient science, Vastu Shastra has developed into a comprehensive architectural concept used to design aesthetically pleasing and energy-inviting buildings to encourage healthy, conscious living. Modern-day Vastu Shastra can be better explained through five fundamental principles:

The 5 Main Principles of Vastu Shastra

1. Site Orientation-Diknirnaya: Directions and How They Are Perceived According to the Principles of Vastu

There is no such thing as a good or bad direction. In the Hindu culture, which is the main source of the Vastu principles, the activities we do in any space must be associated with a specific geographical direction to bolster its effects and bring prosperity. As you'll learn throughout this chapter, directions are the basis upon which all other Vastu principles are built. Unlike standard architects, a Vastu expert would reflect on these considerations before designing any property layout. It isn't just a matter of aesthetics or logical planning. To build a home or office that abounds with good vibes and leads to a happy life, it's imperative to learn the significance of each cardinal direction.

- **North:** This direction is all about career prosperity and material wealth. According to Vastu principles, this direction should be saved for bedrooms, study rooms, and water bodies.

- **South:** This one represents status and prominence. A manager's office or a master bedroom will be conducive to success if built facing the southern orientation.

- **East:** Known as the direction of the sun, the East suggests new beginnings and healing. It's the ideal direction for windows, doors, and gardens. Family rooms can also benefit from the warmth and health properties of this direction.
- **West:** Strength is the dominant quality of the western orientation. A home gym or a study should be built facing west.

Vastu is equally influenced by ordinal directions, detailed below:

- **Northeast:** For mental well-being and feelings of tranquility, pooja rooms and other spiritual activities should be directed toward the northeast. If you've been struggling with your yoga practice and haven't been able to be mindfully present, try changing your location to a northeast-facing space and notice the difference.
- **Northwest:** An airy direction best saved for toilets, bars, and it also works well for kitchens. Guest rooms should face this direction, since it's known as a zone of helpful friends.
- **Southeast:** Also called the zone of Venus, the southeast brings good health and is ideal for kitchens. This direction is equally suitable for spaces dedicated to artistic activities; children's art rooms or home studios can be more inviting and conducive to creativity when in the southeastern zone.
- **Southwest:** Heavy objects should face this direction since it promotes strength. Items like bulky cabinets and overstocked pantries should be facing southeast.

Understanding the meaning behind each direction is only the theoretical aspect of Vastu principles. In practice, you should be able to accurately find each direction in any room. A good way to decide the ideal purpose for a room is to use a compass with your back to its exit and noting the exact orientation. By using this simple technique, you'll be able to easily work out the rest of the directions, both cardinal and ordinal.

2. Site Planning-Vastu Purusha Mandala: How It Relates to Vastu Shastra

One cornerstone of Vastu Shastra is the Vastu Purusha Mandala. In Sanskrit, the word Mandala literally means "circle." The term can also refer to any diagram that can be a guiding tool in any endeavor, be it spiritual or architectural, as is the case here with Vastu Shastra. Historically, Vastu Purusha Mandala first came about when Brahma promised its namesake monster a prayer every time a man builds a structure on Earth to compensate for his suffering after Brahma pinned him down and left him incapacitated. The Vastu Shastra Mandala diagram depicted this tale and was a reference point for the principles of Vastu Shastra. Legend has it there were 45 gods pinning down the monster Vastu Purusha, and their positioning influenced the significance of each of the cardinal and ordinal directions. Each god had their unique powers and represented unique qualities. For example, as you'll learn later in this chapter, the center of any structure should be kept wide open since the supreme Brahma was the one occupying the center of the Vastu Purusha Mandala. Angi, the lord of fire, was occupying the southeast direction, which associated it with passion and creativity.

3. Proportions of The Building-Maana

The right ratio between height and breadth must be respected for optimum functionality and a pleasant overall look to design effective and harmonious structures. The energetic balance element cannot be overlooked because, after all, Vastu is all about achieving this coveted objective. For many years, Vastu scholars worked hard to identify the perfect measurements to act as a guide for anyone who wishes to erect a well-proportioned building. Eventually, they named a set of ideal ratios of height to breadth that can be applied universally:

- A building with its height equal to its breadth is considered proportionate
- A building with its height 1.25 times the size of its breadth is said to be adequately stable

- A building with its height 1.5 times the size of its breadth is pleasant to look at
- A building with its height 1.75 times the size of its breadth is sturdy and beautiful
- A building with its height two times the size of its breadth is optimal

Abiding by the abovementioned construction ratios will guarantee balance, harmony, and consistency in neighborhoods and cities; they are ideal for creating proportionate and aesthetically pleasing structures and living communities in any urban setting.

4. Dimensions of The Building-Aayadi

A principle of Vastu Shastra identifies six essential formulas for deciding on the height, length, width, parameter, and area when designing a building to make sure it ends up beautiful. It goes as follows:

- The Yoni and Vyaya formulas can enhance the breadth
- The Aaya, Vyaya, and Raksha can enhance the length
- The Yoni formula can also fix the orientation of a building that wasn't initially designed with the cardinal directions in mind.

5. Aesthetics of The Building-Chanda

Chanda, which translates to 'beauty,' refers to a building's aesthetics. Vastu is a science that respects proportionality and logic. However, this comprehensive architectural system also minds the element of beauty and how a structure should appease both onlookers and dwellers. The Chanda principle makes it easier to identify different buildings far away according to their function and purpose. For instance, all temples were essentially shaped like mountains and are easy to locate. There are four main types of Vastu Chandas that can be used with building. These include:

- **Meru Chanda:** As seen on many Hindu temples, in Meru Chanda, buildings have a long, pointed top

• **Khanda Meru Chanda:** Here, the building doesn't have a uniform outwardly shape
• **Pataaka Chanda:** Buildings with a Pataaka Chanda resemble a bird's wings spread wide open
• **Sushi Chanda:** In Sushi Chanda, a building has a needle-like pointed tip

What is Pancha Bhoota?

According to Vastu, elements are of paramount importance; each believed to inhibit a specific direction. As explained earlier, in the Vedic tradition, there are five elements in nature: earth, water, fire, air, and space. Each element represents a facet of human life, which, if kept in balance, will promote Zen, healthy, and prosperous living. Below, we analyze the importance of categorizing the activities you do and the objects that surround you to understand how you can combine directions and elements for optimum results:

• **Earth:** Heavy objects that share the yellow and brown shades of soil and stones are considered earthy items. For instance, a chest of drawers made of wood or a stone sculpture is earthy objects, and they're best paired with the southwestern direction that will promote stability and grounding.

• **Water:** Humans have revered water since the dawn of time. This fundamental element symbolizes the essence of life and continuity. Vastu postulates that flowing water represents fluidity and avoiding stagnation. Remembering that, it's easy to see that with architecture and design, you'd want to locate any body of water (an indoor fountain or a swimming pool) in the northern wing of your home to heighten their effects.

- **Fire:** Fire is the element associated with power and influence. Matching your fireplace, stove, and other fiery elements with the south, this direction of prominence will intensify the positive effects in your home.

- **Air:** If you've ever wondered why an easy-going and pleasant person is described as "airy," it's because the air element is all about happiness and lightness. This element resides in the east, and when combined with its original inhabitant, the sun, it can bring about immense joy and an abundance of luck. When building your new home, doors and windows should always face east to keep the air element well-balanced.

- **Space:** Space is the element of central areas and signifies constant improvement. It's crucial to make way for energy to flow freely at the center of any place. The west direction is the recommended one for space elements. A foyer or a large hallway in an office should be kept clutter-free, and preferably with a high and sunlit ceiling for maximum positive energy.

While the information can seem overwhelming, with time, you'll be able to categorize objects around you into elements and find the perfect spot to place them. You can always use this book as a reference guide whenever you're confused about how to best combine different elements and directions in your home or office space.

The Importance of Colors in Accordance with Vastu Shastra

In Vastu Shastra, colors also play a dynamic role and are considered one of the essential principles of this science and art. You cannot possibly build a Vastu-compliant space without grasping the idea behind each color to be utilized in the best way possible. Different colors reflect different energies and are best paired with specific directions and rooms in any home. But since we all have our own preferences, there isn't a rigid, unified Vastu color code. Instead, we will discuss the main colors and generally show you how you can best use them:

- **Blue:** Blue is a color of relaxation and serenity. Since it's associated with water bodies, its properties can come to life in the northeastern direction. Painting a room a soothing shade of blue will help instill a feeling of calmness and relaxation. However, if blue walls do not match your room's theme, try adding blue accents instead. You can accessorize the room with blue décor items, cushions, or hang turquoise frames on the wall. Find the amount of blue that you're comfortable with, yet don't miss out on the amazing qualities of this iconic color.

- **Green:** The green color is perfect for promoting healing energy. Walls in hospitals and retirement homes are usually painted in therapeutic shades of green. According to Vastu, the north is the direction that works best with green. Using indoor plants can also capture the green color's healing powers if you've already chosen to go with neutral-colored walls.

- **Yellow:** Yellow is a happy color that is more impactful when used toward creativity, which is the southeast. Save this color for your kids' bedroom to spark joy and in your kitchen to emphasize the warmth in this cozy space.

- **Pink:** Pink denotes love, and when used in a southeast-facing room, can help improve intimacy and closeness between its occupants. Since pink is often stereotyped as "girly," you can choose pink accessories rather than paint an entire wall in pink.

- **Purple:** Purple is an omen of wealth and prosperity. It suits the south direction and can ease feelings of anxiety and depression.

• **Brown:** Last, brown and beige tones are the ultimate earthy colors. As one would expect, they come across particularly well in the southwest direction where the earth element resides. Under Vastu, using brown shades effectively brings stability and balance to any space.

Vastu Shastra is a wholesome architectural design philosophy that can be followed from the early inception phases of building. It's a thorough and all-encompassing system that anyone can apply and benefit from. The Vastu essentials that you've just learned in this chapter will come to life over the next chapters, where we will provide concrete actions and steps you can take to build or rearrange a home and workplace under the Vastu precepts.

Chapter 5: Vastu for the Home

Now that you understand more about Vastu Shastra and how it can help create an environment of prosperity and abundance in living spaces, it's time to learn how you can achieve it. This chapter will dig deeper into Vastu Shastra design precepts and give you plenty of ideas on how to incorporate them harmoniously and effectively. Whether your home is still in its conception or construction phase, or if you've inhabited it for a while, you can greatly benefit from the concepts of Vastu. And while Vastu Shastra can be applied in any space, this chapter's focus will be on the home since it's where people spend most of their time.

First: Applying Vastu Shastra During Construction

Starting with a clean slate will grant you a better chance to incorporate The Vastu principles into every corner of your house. Generally, all the rooms should be square or rectangular, with four cornered ceilings to attract abundance and joy. Here, we discuss how to use simple tips to make every room in your house Vastu-compliant. Let's get started!

- ### Choose the Entrance Direction Wisely

  As per the Vastu science, the sun is considered the main source of positive energy. Directing your home entrance towards the east, where the sun rises will set you out on a great track to start. If you choose not to work with a specialized Vastu consultant, meet with your contractor before building the rest of the house. Given that your entrance is the main gateway for outside energy to penetrate your space, you need this to be a 'good door' to invite prosperity and keep away the negative vibes. Choosing teak wood for your entrance door can attract even more positivity. If you aren't building your own home and looking for a ready-to-move property, it's best to remember that and focus on finding a house with an east-facing entryway. Avoid property with an entrance facing southwest, since this is said to be the entrance of evil energy that carries struggles and hardships to the home dwellers. A southeast entrance is not any good either, as it's believed to be a direction that lets in sickness and anger.

• Find the Perfect Location For Your Kitchen

When choosing where to place your kitchen, Vastu teachings recommend a southeast direction for auspiciousness. In addition, the location of the kitchen in your house is just as important. You cannot have the kitchen facing a bathroom or a bedroom. For a propitious kitchen, walls should be painted in a bright color, like green or red, to create a pleasing aura. During construction, have at least a couple of windows in your kitchen since open windows let good energy in. Also, installing an exhaust fan will allow the room to ventilate and let the negative energy out. If you're leaning towards built-in electrical appliances, you must think about the placement of each. For the stove, which represents the fire element, it must be facing a southeast direction. But the sink is a water element that should be placed nowhere near its fire nemesis; a northeast direction works better for easy water-flowing. As for the refrigerator, place it facing a southwest direction, away from any corners.

• Build Your Bedroom in the South Western Corners

With the most important room in your house, namely the bedroom, be careful about its placement. Your bedroom is supposed to be your sanctuary, where you get to relax and rest after a long and exhausting day. A southwest corner is ideal for your bedroom to make sure you don't pave the way for the disrupting "agni" energy that governs the southeast, which promotes misunderstanding and violence between couples. Also, dedicate one of the southwestern facing walls to your cupboard, and make sure that they open towards the north to promote the flow of positive energy throughout the room. Ask your contractor to leave enough space for your bedroom door to open at a 90-degree angle; this makes way for prosperous opportunities for the occupants. Ideally, the walls should be painted in neutral and soothing shades of pink, blue, or gray.

• Have a Spacious Hallway

According to The Vastu principles, the center of the home is believed to be its beating heart. When planning your house's layout, include a spacious hallway in its center. As the place where all energies come together and their powers reach their peaks, you must create a pathway for the positive ones to come in and the bad ones to flow out. This will create a beautiful, pacifying harmony throughout.

• Build the Perfect Pooja Room

Since a pooja room is where you will be meditating and praying, you must think carefully about how you can optimize the good energies in there. Vastu Shastra precepts recommend avoiding basements or top floors for your pooja room; the ground floor is the optimum choice for this sacred spot. Also, the northeast orientation is the favored direction for your pooja room. If you have enough space, ask your contractor to account for a 2-door entryway and a threshold to keep ants and other bugs out of your sacred room. Similarly, plan to have a low pyramid-shaped ceiling for symmetry that will help you achieve a meditative state with ease. As far as selecting a color scheme for the pooja room, choose bright and serene colors that are peaceful to look at (pearl white, cream, pastels). Don't forget to install storage cabinets facing southeast to keep your pooja books and incense bundles neatly organized.

• **Select the Right Location For Your Bathrooms**

A bathroom shouldn't be built next to or facing your kitchen. Instead, it should be in the northwest or southeast corners of the house. Bathroom doors should be placed along northern or eastern walls. Don't only think about convenience and décor when deciding where to locate the bathroom fixtures. Toilets should ideally be placed a few inches above the ground; floating toilets are trendier anyway, so you shouldn't have a problem finding ones that will complement the aesthetics and spiritual value of your house. While on toilet bowl placements, it should be placed along the west or northwestern walls of the bathroom as it symbolizes waste-discarding. Just like your bedroom, Vastu principles encourage using light pastel colors in your bathrooms, such as light blues, grays, or plain white.

• **Pay Attention To Your Kids' Room**

Your kids' room should teem with warmth and love to encourage their development and growth. When you are first designing its layout, it's important to remember some important facts. The door to the bedroom should be clockwise to keep away the negative energy responsible for sibling fights and rivalry. Their beds should be facing no windows, doors, or mirrors. Just like in your room, best to keep mirrors away from the beds to avoid the reflection of bad energies. If you are placing bookshelves inside the bedroom, they should face northeast and be made from warm, auspicious material like wood. It's also a smart idea to have your contractor design custom built-in cabinets and extra storage solutions for your kids to keep their room clutter-free and avoid disrupting energy flow. However, don't be tempted to add a storage unit under their beds. According to Vastu principles, this can induce nightmares and disrupt prosperity. If your kids are old enough, consider involving them in building a Vastu-compliant home. This will encourage them and teach them the importance of keeping their rooms always tidy and clean.

Second: Vastu Shastra For Your Current Home

To reap the benefits of Vastu in your existing home, there are essentials you can incorporate for impeccable results. These are:

• Add Bamboo For a Healthy Life

In Hinduism, plants are a symbol of health and good fortune, especially Bamboo, a sign of vitality and well-being for centuries. Invariably, bamboo plants are a must-have for any home that follows the basics of Vastu. But there are guidelines for putting this lucky plant on display. Foremost, as an indoor plant, green bamboo poles best thrive away from direct sunlight, so place your bamboo plant in a see-through glass container in the eastern corner of the room. For ultimate prosperity, try to combine the five elements (water, metal, fire, earth, and wood). Adding a red-colored fiery ribbon on the wooden bamboo poles makes two of the elements, to which you can then add stones and coins in the water-filled vase to tie all the elements together. Make sure the bamboo poles are always well-watered and kept fresh; wilting bamboos can bring bad luck and misfortune upon a home's occupants.

• Having a Buddha Statue on Display

Regardless of your religious beliefs, if you have any in the first place, Buddha is a respected figure believed to signify prosperity and good luck. According to Vastu's science, placing Buddha figurines made of bronze has the power to attract positive energy into your house and ward off negativity and harmful energies. Even if your décor isn't necessarily oriental, Buddha figurines are always a nice addition, and they won't seem out of place when you feel their strong effects.

• Turtle Figurines

In the Hindu tradition, turtles are a symbol of longevity, which mirrors these reptiles' impressive lifespan. According to the Vastu precepts, decorating your family room with metal or mud turtle figurines will bring good luck and happy and lengthy life.

• Pay Homage to Ganesha

Ganesha, the god of luck in Hinduism, is considered a sacred figure for anyone who believes in the powers of Vastu Shastra. You can pay homage to Ganesha as you prefer. However, it's recommended to place the Ganesha statue in your home's entryway and on top of an elevated structure, such as a floating shelf or a marble column. If you have an extra room you dedicate as a spiritual space (like a pooja room), this would be an ideal place for your Ganesha idol. Place it a few inches away from the wall to allow for the energy to flow around it and shower you with its blessings.

• Bowl of Floating Flowers

In most Indian cultures, flowers floating in a bowl of water is considered an unmissable feature in any home. When placed near the home entrance, it sends fortunate wishes towards visiting guests and welcomes them with a pleasant and refreshing smell. Always remember to wash the bowl regularly, change the water, and replace the flowers when they've withered. In doing so, you'll be inviting good vibes into your abode and checking an additional box for a Vastu-compliant home.

• A Fish Tank

According to Vastu teachings, aquariums have the power to reverse the negative effects caused by Vastu defects. Such defects occur when people disregard the importance of an objects placement or the energy flow of their home. A fish tank placed in a southeastern direction should reverse these undesirable effects and promote harmony.

Ultimately, those are important tenets of Vastu Shastra you must remember when building, furnishing, and decorating your home. In parallel, you can incorporate several essential daily habits to make it fully Vastu-compliant. Here's a quick and practical run-through to achieve a harmonious and balanced life at home:

• Keep your entrance clear to avoid disrupting the flow of good energy. If you don't want to regularly pick up your kids' shoes, install a shoe closet to optimize the space, and make your life easier.

• Display Vastu-friendly art. Images of flowing rivers, fish, and waterfalls are all Vastu paintings that attract wealth and auspiciousness into your life. If living abroad is a dream of yours, you can express this by hanging paintings of flying birds or photographs of trains and cars around your house.

• With financial prosperity, Vastu principles suggest hanging wind chimes at the entrance of your home. Alternatively, you can place them at the entrance of your bathroom to trap in wealth and prevent its escape. But you should never place wind chimes anywhere around your bedroom, as this can summon unfavorable negative effects, such as illness and misfortune.

• Maintaining clocks around your home in good condition is believed to attract wealth and pave the way for lucrative ventures.

• Feeding birds is not only a kind act, but it's also one practice you can implement for Vastu Shastra. Placing a simple bird feeder on your porch or balcony will make the birds come flocking your way, bringing along all the good luck and prosperity.

• Where you place mirrors around your house can make a world of difference in the energy you attract. According to The Vastu principles, having a mirror over your bed will reflect negative energy and hinder prosperity. A mirror above your chest of drawers where you keep your valuable items can help grow your wealth.

• Using purple orchids, pots, and linens to decorate your home is one of the simplest ways for maintaining the flow of good energy throughout your home. Purple is the color of health and wisdom, which means the more you incorporate it into your life, the more it will pay you back in health and auspiciousness.

• Ventilating your bedroom by letting in fresh air and sunshine will cleanse your home's aura and prepare you to receive wealth and good luck. As such, it makes it a habit to open the windows every day to allow the air to flow through, bringing in the positive energy and evacuating the negative one. Even during cold winter months, you keep up this practice, even for a few minutes during the morning and evening. You're bound to feel an instant mood lift by breathing in the fresh air, both before and after a good night's rest.

• If you've been struggling with bad luck for a while and you're ready to turn that around, light one lamp beside your bowl of floating flowers or aquarium each night.

• Last, make sure the toilet cover is always always down and the bathroom door closed.

As you can see, there are countless ways through which you can instill a more Vastu-friendly home living. Even if the concepts seem foreign to western architecture and interior design, try for yourself to see how different your life will be when you carry out these Vastu principles. Don't be overwhelmed by the information and recommendations listed above. The beauty of Vastu is that you can start small, and once you understand the reasoning behind each of its basic concepts, you'll be ready for bigger changes. In the next chapter, we'll move on to the workplace and provide valuable insight on how to use the science and art of Vastu to turn your office into a space conducive to productivity, wealth, and prosperity.

Chapter 6: Vastu for the Workplace

As a business owner, you may be wondering about how Vastu Shastra relates to business. The guidelines the system offers are not just limited to residential areas, but they can also be used in offices, factories, hotels, or any other business venue. Applying the precepts of Vastu Shastra to the organization of your workplace can help you generate more profits, ensure harmony, and stem the negative flow of energy in it. In this chapter, you'll find easy-to-follow tips on how you can use Vastu Shastra to propel your business forward.

The Benefits of Vastu Shastra for Business

While Vastu Shastra on its own isn't a magical solution to all your business woes, following its principles can alleviate stress you and your team might be under. Since implementing the teachings of Vastu Shastra may entail changing the whole organization of your workplace, it only makes sense you might be interested in knowing more about the benefits you will reap by doing so. If you're interested in employing the rules of this art in your work area, check out these reasons why this is considered a worthwhile investment.

Achieving Clarity

In business, you always must be quick on your feet and adapt to changing market demands if you want your venture to thrive. Naturally, this is easier said than done. Making split-second decisions while ensuring that they serve your company's interests is more challenging than it sounds. Therefore, most business owners strive to achieve clarity, as this allows them to weigh their options quickly and come up with the best solution without dwelling on matters too much or crumbling under pressure. Vastu Shastra is a sure-fire way of achieving clarity because it eradicates the flow of negative energy and provides you with the focus and support you need for your business goals.

Generating More Income

Truth be told, money is always at the forefront of everyone's mind, and you'd be lying if you claimed otherwise. Finding ways to generate more profits is also something that many business owners put in a lot of time and effort into. What if we told you that you could double or even triple your income just by implementing Vastu Shastra in your workplace? Far from being unfounded superstitions, the precepts of Vastu Shastra will put your company on the right track, increasing its opportunities for scaling up and attracting more clients. Whether you have a shop or own a factory, you're bound to notice a considerable increase in your sales when you apply the teachings of this science to your work environment.

Inspiring Your Team

Work is hard and keeping your team of collaborators motivated can turn into a herculean task if you don't know what you're doing. Although there are countless tips online and productivity books that cover several methods of enhancing creativity and motivation in professional settings, they are never effective if not coupled with the teachings of Vastu Shastra. If you apply these tips without keeping the principles of Vastu Shastra in mind, you'll be basically disregarding the root of the problem, namely negative energy. The best way to boost workplace productivity is to look for the problem area and remedy it right away, and this can be done only by implementing Vastu Shastra. This art enables people to be more in sync with their souls and allows them to draw on the surrounding inspiration to come up with more creative and valuable ideas.

Eliminating Discord

Workplace quarrels are common, regardless of the scale of your company or the size of your team. Such fights are almost always accompanied by dips in production and sales, plus they create a negative work environment where people are not comfortable voicing their opinions. Even if your staff members are always in sync with each other, they might still feel stressed out, especially if their jobs involve sitting in front of a computer all day. Because these jobs usually make people restless and more prone to irritability, you must continuously find ways to bring your team together. To enhance the harmony in your company, consider applying the principles of Vastu Shastra. From the choice of color palette and lighting to furniture placement, Vastu Shastra covers all the essentials you need to give your staff a positive, inspiring, and supportive work environment.

General Vastu Shastra Rules for Business

Considering the abundance of benefits, Vastu Shastra entails, you might be now interested in learning how you can apply its teachings to your business. Before we delve deep into these principles, you can implement in the workplace, you need to know some of the dos and don'ts of business as per Vastu Shastra's basic tenets. These can be summarized as follows:

Do's

- Always make sure that you have a wall behind your desk because it fosters support. You can reinforce this further by adding pictures of mountains, which symbolize stability and strength.

• Declutter the area in front of your desk to create a sense of openness and trust.

• Pick only wooden furniture

• Get high-back chairs. They are not only great for your back, but they also denote support.

• Place plants and lamps in the southeastern part of your workspace to increase your wealth and career growth

• Keep your workplace well-lit to dispel negative energy.

• Fix or replace broken furniture and faucets right away because keeping them in such a state will induce negative energy.

Don'ts

• Don't hang pictures of water or fluids on the wall behind your desk, as this will undermine your support. Likewise, avoid any pictures illustrating crying people, violence, struggle, etc.

• Don't cross your legs because this repels growth opportunities.

• Don't buy furniture that comes in irregular shapes: circular, triangular, oval, etc. Instead, stick to sturdy square-shaped or rectangular pieces.

• Vastu Shastra for Offices

• If you have limited office space, it may be wise to use Vastu Shastra to optimize the place and bring in more clients. Following are some rules you can follow to make sure that your office does not exude negative energy.

Office Location

We've already mentioned how irregularly shaped plots of land attract negative energy. Now, if you still do not have an office, make sure that the area you're considering is rectangular or square. The office should also be in a populous area to increase prosperity and your staff's productivity, so steer away from establishing your workplace off the beaten track. Offices should face east because positive energy flows in this direction, which will make your business more prosperous. If you plan on adding a drinking fountain or any other water source, it should be kept in the northeast, as this is the direction of the element of water. Generally, avoid having stairs or any other obstructions in the middle of the office. As explained in an earlier chapter, this area should be left empty to allow the energy to circulate effortlessly.

To add mirrors, make sure that they are placed in the northern section of the office to help you generate more income. They play a big role in Vastu Shastra; offices should be painted in bright colors to promote liveliness and enthusiasm.

Where You Should Sit

You are the head of operations, and ensure that your desk is ideally placed. Business owners and managers should always face north when dealing with clients since the north is the direction of the deity Kuber, the lord of wealth. North also denotes career advancement. Therefore, as a business owner, you should make sure that your desk faces this orientation. Don't sit under beams because they support the whole structure; sitting under them can negatively affect your fortune, making it harder to bring in and finalize new deals. Also, avoid seating arrangements that cause your back to face doors because this can create an ambiance of mistrust. To foster support, make sure that you always have a wall behind you. If you work from home, make sure that your workspace is not next to the master bedroom. Finally, be extra careful about toilet placement by keeping them in the north or northwestern area of the office, just like you would at home.

Where Your Staff and Clients Should Sit

Keep your staff on the eastern side of the office, as the east is the direction of prosperity. The northeast is the direction of wealth and growth. You should make sure that your company's reception desk faces the northeast. Avoid putting any fire element in this direction, as it can cause accidents and attract bad luck. If you have waiting rooms, they should be in the northeast or northwest, which are the natural directions of water and air. This will reinforce the clients' patience by supplying them with a large dose of positive energy.

Vastu Shastra for Factories

If you own a factory or are building one, the following are the most important Vastu Shastra rules to remember.

Factory Placement

When building or buying a factory, make sure it is in the north or east to help increase production and make more profits. Plots of land broader in the front and narrower in the back, known as Shermukhi plots, also bring good luck. Keep the factory entrance in the east, remembering that it must be large enough to establish the flow of positive energy.

Machinery Placement

Your equipment is your real capital. And while accidents happen all the time in factories, you can mitigate this risk thanks to Vastu Shastra. In this spirit, you must place all-electric machinery in the southern or southwestern section of the factory, as these two directions are associated with good health. Keeping equipment in the south and southwest can effectively prevent accidents and common workplace injuries.

Product Placement

You might think that the location of your raw materials, finished merchandise, and inventory does not affect profits or how fast these products sell, but this could not be further from the truth. This is why stacks of raw materials should be kept in the southwest and septic tanks in the north or northwest. When stacking finished products, make sure these piles are placed in the northwestern area. This can help you release the negative energy that might be clinging to them and sell them faster.

Vastu Shastra for Hospitals

If you own or operate a hospital, saving as many lives as possible must be your only priority. Hospitals can harbor an abundance of negative energy, which is why you need to learn how to eliminate negative energy for the safety and wellbeing of your patients. If you're thinking about using Vastu Shastra in your hospital, here are some things you can do:

The Location of the Operation Room

A lot can go wrong during delicate medical procedures, and you must make sure that your operation room is void of any negative energy. With the placement of operation rooms, they should always be in the west. The west is governed by the deity Lord Varun, the god of stability, fate, and rain. By staying under his protection, your patients will have a greater chance of making a stellar recovery. Also, make sure that the operation room entrance is big to attract plenty of positive energy.

Ventilation

Adequate ventilation is not only good for patients' health, but it can also expel negative energy. You should always keep your patient's room well ventilated. This can be done by adding large-width doors or windows. However, be careful about placing these windows, lest you invite in more negative energy! As a rule of thumb, windows should be placed in the east, the direction most associated with the sun element.

Equipment Placement

Extensive medical knowledge is not the only thing that factors in patients' health and recovery. Ensuring that the hospital's equipment is in tip-top shape can also go a long way towards achieving this end, which is why the institution's storage solutions should reflect this. Just like factory machinery, medical equipment must be kept at ground level in the west or southwest to prevent accidents or malfunctions.

Recovery Room Placement

Guaranteeing speedy recovery is something that doctors typically care a great deal about. With Vastu Shastra, you can help your patients get back on their feet and enjoy precious moments with their families much faster. When setting up recovery rooms, make sure that they are in the southwestern portion of the hospital; this direction is strongly linked to good health and is governed by the demon Niriti and planet Rahu.

The Placement of Your Office

We've already covered how Vastu Shastra can be used to provide improved health for your patients, but what about your health? Rest assured, as the teachings of Vastu Shastra can also be beneficial for doctors, nurses, and hospital owners. If you can choose your office's location, always pick north or east because these directions can increase the flow of power and success. As always, avoid any irregularly shaped furniture and make sure that the room itself is rectangular or square-shaped. By doing so, you will attract many opportunities to prove your competence and further your career.

Vastu Shastra for Shops

Due to the spread of COVID-19, running a brick-and-mortar shop has become increasingly challenging. With social distancing rules and limitations to remember, you may not have enough time or resources to dedicate to implementing the principles of Vastu Shastra in your commercial business. But not only can Vastu Shastra help your shop stand out and catch the eye of more people, but it will also enhance its prosperity and longevity. However, check out the next few tips to learn how you can make your shop Vastu-compliant.

The General Organization of the Place

When you're renovating your shop, you may disregard the rules of Vastu Shastra for improving the overall aesthetic of the place. Although, this is a fatal mistake that can ruin your business, it's potential for growth and impact your profits. To add extensions to the shop, make sure not to alter the rectangular or square shape of the place because, as you're well aware by now, irregular shapes function as magnets of bad luck and negative vibes. And stack your product in neat piles and place them in the northwestern section of the shop. Also keep the entrance in the east or northeast to make the place more inviting. Regularly check to make sure that the doors do not squeak, as this can increase the flow of inauspicious energy. Your cash counter should be carefully installed so it allows it to open towards the north, the direction of the deity Kuber, the god of wealth. Finally, if you dabble in electronics, e.g., computers, televisions, phones, etc., keep these products in the southeast instead of the northwest.

Ultimately, the teachings of Vastu Shastra can be applied to all walks of life, including business. No matter your occupation or position in your company's hierarchy, the tips in this chapter will be of great help in furthering your career and leading a fuller, more prosperous life. Whether you want to seek help from a Vastu consultant or reorganize your work area yourself, make sure not to disregard the principles of Vastu Shastra because this might bring about adverse effects in the long run.

Chapter 7: Design Principles: Architecture and Interior Designing

Vastu Shastra might seem like an outdated concept. It's been around for thousands of years, and what might have worked eons ago doesn't apply to modern architecture. This also explains why many people are reluctant to implement Vastu design precepts in their work or living spaces. Regardless of what uninformed individuals may believe, Vastu Shastra still bears incredible significance today. In this chapter, you'll discover the benefits of this art in modern architecture, along with quick tips on how to apply its principles for more harmony and prosperity.

Why Is Vastu Shastra Still Relevant Today?

Even if you strongly believe in the ancient science of Vastu Shastra, it still might be hard to justify implementing its teachings in the 21st century. It also doesn't help that balancing its teachings and modern interior design trends can be challenging and costly. There are two different opinions. Architects believe that Vastu Shastra is just an old paradigm that holds little merit nowadays. But others think that Vastu can still be integrated into modern architecture despite being an old science. The second group seems to have it right, though. Since Vastu Shastra is based on Earth's magnetic field principles, cardinal directions, natural elements, and Prana (the Earth's energy), it qualifies as a powerful tool for achieving harmonious living. These elements are timeless, so they still affect us to varying degrees. Because such powers virtually haven't changed one bit throughout the years, you still need to heed the teachings of Vastu Shastra to stay protected and ward off negative energy. Therefore, we're inclined to say this art has not withered by time but has only grown even more vital.

Why Should Vastu Shastra Be Integrated into Modern Architecture?

Saying that art is still today usually isn't enough to incentivize people to try it. When money is a factor, most property owners should learn more about the concrete benefits before investing a dime in something. Now, if you're still on the fence about Vastu Shastra, here are reasons integrating its principles into modern architecture is well worth it.

Vastu Shastra Encourages Optimal Use of Space

Let's forget about Vastu's spiritual aspect for a while and think about how it can save you a pretty penny! While true that changing an already-established space to make it Vastu-compliant can be an arduous task sometimes, you'd be surprised at how much money it can save you. If you're thinking about up sizing to a bigger office or house, it might be wise to analyze how you're using the space you already have. Usually people who don't follow Vastu Shastra's principles end up with cluttered spaces that barely have enough room for their furniture and belongings. With Vastu, you'll be able to make the best use of any space, not just by decluttering it but by organizing it so it allows for more expansion, which is always a plus, especially for business owners. By integrating this philosophy into interior design, you may realize that there's to move to a bigger house after all! That's quite a bit of saving, to say the least.

Vastu Shastra Is Easy to Implement

Given the many rules, Vastu Shastra has, implementing them may feel like you've bitten more than you can chew. With countless factors and placement strategies to remember, applying Vastu Shastra to your living or work area might seem downright impractical. But don't knock it until you try it! Vastu Shastra sounds like a complicated concept, especially to those who've never heard about it before. However, once you understand its core rules, implementing it becomes child's play. It all boils down to following its guidelines. Fortunately, Vastu Shastra's design principles haven't changed for millennia, which means you'll easily find plenty of professionals willing to help if you still believe you cannot handle it on your own.

Vastu Shastra Brings Financial Gains and Emotional Stability

Life is admittedly hard at the moment. With a pandemic on the rise, saving a few pennies here and there can make all the difference. What if we told you there was an easy way to markedly improve your financial situation? While applying the principles of Vastu Shastra isn't a guaranteed way of becoming wealthy, it does open many doors. Financial gain is one of the greatest benefits associated with this science. By encouraging the flow of positive energy, you'll reap many merits this comes with, including monetary ones. You're also bound to find yourself more at ease in a Vastu-compliant space. Since Vastu's main goals are to curtail the flow of negative energy, you'll let go of grudges and feel more satisfied with your life.

Vastu Shastra Builds Trust and Harmony

Whether you have a big family or run a business, you know how tension can get to people and make them fight over the silliest of things. Although many people think that quarrels among siblings and work colleagues are normal, have you thought about why they happen in the first place? Naturally, many of these misunderstandings can be attributed to ego or stress, but you cannot discount the energy that permeates the places where such arguments start. Places filled with negative vibes make people more irritable, quicker to jump to conclusions, and blame others. This is simply the result of ignoring the teachings of Vastu. The only way to remedy this is to investigate integrating Vastu Shastra into modern architecture.

Vastu Shastra Tips for Modern Architecture

Choosing Sites

To start implementing the principles of Vastu Shastra, start with the ones that relate to how you can choose auspicious sites. These are:

Soil

From a scientific perspective, the quality of the soil determines how strong a building's foundations are. Whether you're an architect or a would-be property owner, you must keep this rule in mind to choose a suitable, future-proof plot of land. When on the market for land, pick a plot with cultivable soil, even if you don't plan to grow crops once you buy it. The color of the soil itself can help you decide whether it is cultivable or not. Yellow, brown, and brick red soil are generally considered good for planting crops, whereas black and clay-like soil aren't. Now, how does the color of the soil or its potential for cultivability affect a building's foundations? Clay-like and black soil holds excess moisture, which can weaken the foundations of your property. Uncultivable soil also doesn't allow for good drainage, causing foundations to debilitate as time passes. Rocky soil, too, is a bad choice because you must pay extra to make it suitable for laying your foundations. Sites that are teeming with worms or have graves are off-limits as per the teachings of Vastu Shastra. Not only do these sites increase the flow of negative energy, but they also signal that the soil itself is loose, meaning it will not offer enough stability and support for your foundations.

Is there another way to assess the quality of the soil without depending on its color? Yes, there are two simple tests you can try to see if the soil is good enough as a base for your building. First, you can try digging a small hole, 2 x 2 x 2 inches, and fill it with water. After an hour, check whether the soil has absorbed the water. If excess water is left, this is a sign that the soil is perfect for construction. But if the soil absorbs all the water in an hour or less or becomes all cracked up, it means that it's either too loose or too clay-like; this indicates that the land isn't ideal for construction. The second test involves digging a hole with the same afore-mentioned dimensions and then refilling it. If you refill the hole completely, whether you end up with excess soil or not, then the location is suitable for construction. But if you run out of the soil before refilling the hole completely, this suggests that the soil is too dense and holds excess moisture easily.

Site Orientation

According to the Vastu Purusha Mandala, designing spaces is easier when the orientation of the site itself is optimal. However, in Vastu Shastra, there is no particularly "evil" or "auspicious" direction; it all depends on the purpose of the building. Sites that face Purva (east) are best suited for schools and universities, as this direction provides enlightenment, making it the best for those constantly pursuing knowledge. Spots that face Uttara (north) are ideal for governmental buildings or any other structures reserved for those in positions of power, such as presidents, ministers, or congresspeople. But Dakshina-facing (south-facing) locations are usually used for commercial businesses. Finally, sites facing (west) are left for facilities that supply people with miscellaneous services. Buildings established in locations facing the cardinal directions recognized by Vastu Shastra will provide the people living or working in them with the benefits of being in sync with the natural elements. For architects, it is crucial to choose the right location when establishing residential or commercial buildings to make sure that the site itself is Vastu-compliant.

Location

The location of any property, whether residential or commercial, is the first thing you should be concerned about when you're on the market for one. Ideally, go for plenty of lush greenery areas, as this is a sign of prosperity. Never overlook the history of the property; violence often leaves an imprint, so avoid properties sold by people in distress because the negative energy they've left behind will be transferred to you, causing you to be constantly on edge and ready to pick arguments. Properties, where people committed suicide or homicide are also a big no-no. You don't want to risk dealing with the negative imprint such tragic events leave in their wake.

If you're looking for a house, make sure that it's in a residential area. Living close to public places, such as schools, hospitals, and temples, goes against the rules of Vastu Shastra. Don't buy plots of land relatively smaller compared to the ones near it. Unconsciously, you might feel like you are less fortunate than your neighbors if you choose such a property setup. Properties blocked from the eastern direction by larger buildings are also considered inauspicious, as they get little natural sunlight. The same applies to habitations that have power supply stations in the northeastern direction. These stations create an "obstruction," which blocks the flow of positive energy and permeates the place with negative vibes.

In parallel, you must also be careful about the roads surrounding the property. Plots of land that face roads in the northeast are considered auspicious because this means that the northern part of the property is open, which is an important rule in Vastu Shastra. Finally, steer away from buildings or plots of land that face Y or T intersections (Veedi Shoolas). Veedi Shoolas draw negative energy, dust, and wind to the place, plus they considerably undermine your privacy. But if you've come across a great property that faces a Veedi Shoola, you can still make tweaks that will help you deflect the negative energy emanating from the intersection. For example, you can turn the part facing the road into a garage or a parking area. Using big trees or convex mirrors to block the intersection's negative energy is also an effective solution. If all fails, you can fence off that area. In any case, follow your intuition. If the place feels uncomfortable, simply continue your search for another property. Don't brush aside these feelings as pure superstition, as your body and soul know when they're not in sync with the elements. It's important to heed their warning.

Quick Vastu-Compliant Interior Design Tips

So, you've made sure that the location of your building and its orientation is Vastu-compliant, now what? Of course, it's time to tweak your interior design! Here's how you can follow Vastu Shastra's principles and ensure that your property retains its modern vibe:

- The main entrance of the building should face east or north and be made from high-quality wood. It should also open in a clockwise manner and be bigger than any other door the building has. Finally, don't paint it black or any other dark color or place garbage cans near it because this repels positive energy.
- If the building has a pooja or meditation room, use green and yellow for the walls and add incense sticks to repel negative energy. Avoid red because it indicates anger. Ideally, this room should face northeast or east.
- If a room includes electric appliances, they should be kept in the southwestern or western portion.
- Avoid including irregularly shaped furniture in any area, as it increases the flow of negative energy.
- Always keep the premises well-lit.
- Make sure that you're not facing any mirrors for extended periods. This entails removing mirrors placed in front of beds or couches. Mirrors are usually used to attract and lock in negative energy, protecting the place's residents

from stumbling upon it. Although, staring too long in a mirror can make this energy reflect onto you. Also, avoid sitting with your back facing reflective surfaces.

• Remove any graffiti on the outside walls of the building, as it can bring chaos into your life if not tended to.

• Rooms where people congregate, such as living and meeting rooms, should be painted in yellow, white, blue, or green. Black and dark tones should generally be avoided.

• Colors like peach, pink, light green, blue, and orange can be used for cafeterias, dining rooms, and restaurants.

• Spaces that include the element of fire, such as kitchens, should be painted in fiery red, bright yellow, or orange to pay homage to Agni, the god of fire. Steer clear of dark tones to reduce the flow of negative energy, and shades of blue, because it's the color of the god of water, Varuna.

• Rest areas, including bedrooms and break rooms, can be painted in either blue and green for relaxation or brown for stability. If you and your partner recently got married, you can use colors like red and light pink to signify passion and intimacy. To increase productivity, you can try incorporating orange into the design of the room. Be careful, though, since people can get quickly agitated because of this color!

As we've seen, incorporating Vastu Shastra's principles in modern architecture and interior design isn't as complex as it sounds. While you may think that you must sacrifice the modern ambiance of your property to apply Vastu's teachings. I hope you now know how easy it is. Most important, don't listen to those who try to undersell Vastu Shastra as an outdated concept. This science is *very much* alive and well!

Chapter 8: Integrating Trees and Gardens

As you know by now, trees, plants, and plants make up a large part of Vastu practices. To put together a new garden, you can use the Vastu tips for gardening. Designing a garden from scratch can be an arduous task, as it will require guidance, planning, and consulting with experts to get the best results. Luckily, traditional Vastu guides for planting trees and designing gardens will alleviate that confusion and considerably facilitate this green endeavor. In this chapter, we'll explain how you can employ Vastu Shastra to create the perfect garden and breathe life into your house so positive energies keep flowing in.

Why are Trees and Plants Important Parts of Vastu?

Generally, the purpose of using Vastu to design your garden is to not only to offer a relaxing and positive environment but also to promote stability and the balance of energies inside and outside your house. Vastu Shastra highlights the importance of plants and greenery, as they're a symbol and embodiment of life. Their placement in the home can help instill serenity and happiness. If you notice that your premise lacks these elements, or if you sense an imbalance in your environment, plant more trees and potted plants. The Vastu charts will clearly show you which types of trees and plants to grow and where you can do that in compliance with auspicious directions.

Choose the Right Location

The first step to consider is the potential location for your new plants. According to Vastu's precepts, five elements exist in your garden, which you must remember for optimal plant and tree placement. While the southwest part of your house represents the earth element, the southeast section stands for fire and is ideal for disease-free plants. The northeast section is a symbol for water, while the northwest represents air. Finally, the center indicates the element of space. Each section will have a different bearing on this area, so plants should be planted according to the garden's location.

East-Facing Houses

Nothing in the Vastu guides indicates that you shouldn't plant trees in an east-facing house. Although, many homeowners have reported this can be considered a bad practice. It's preferable to plant trees on the west side instead; if that's unavoidable, you can create a water sump between the trees and your house to isolate the elements.

West-Facing Houses

If your house faces west, then you're in luck! This orientation is suitable for planting bigger trees. According to Vastu practices, this should avert predicaments and difficult situations for the home's occupants. Strong trees on the west side should help you feel secure and promote success. It should also make your identity more visible, which will help your social life prosper beyond measure.

North-Facing House

Unlike the west, the north direction isn't ideal for massive trees, as this might have adverse effects. Instead, you can choose gardening and planting more compact trees, such as bushes or shrubs. Flowerpots and smaller plants should work in your favor.

South-Facing House

Much like the western direction, the south is an ideal orientation to plant trees and heavy and dense plants. This will have a positive impact on both your health and wealth, as these elements will gravitate toward heavy trees in these areas.

Northeast-Facing House

Since the northeast is associated with a water element, heavy trees (or any tree), it won't be the best option for a garden facing that direction. Ideally, instead opt for grass, small plants, flowers, etc. for landscaping. In that direction, trees' added weight will have a negative effect and should be balanced out with a water sump, as recommended earlier.

Southeast-Facing House

The southeast is another optimal orientation for large and strong trees. If your home is along an east or southeast-facing road, a tree-lined road will dispel negative energies. This will ward off some of the adverse effects from the southwest direction, such as lack of income, bad reputation, and children disputes and rivalries in the household.

Northwest-Facing House

While this direction serves as the element of air, it can be an excellent direction for planting trees. However, to dissipate negative influences, your house's main door must face that direction. This should also be coupled with a naked wall for the home's exterior entrance and ensuring that the number of doors and windows is even.

Southwest-Facing House

Last, since the south and east directions are ideal for placing heavy, bushy trees, planting these same trees in a southwest-facing house is also encouraged. Tall trees in that direction will bring stability and promote a sense of strength. However, fruit-bearing trees are better planted on east-facing houses.

Garden Directions

Helped by these Vastu principles, you'll be able to outfit a beautiful garden from scratch. Before taking on this task, be careful when placing different elements in your garden to repel adverse energy and their spiritually harmful effects. For example, flowerbeds, decorative plants, and lawns should be placed on the garden's north and east sides. Also, to install a cascade or a water feature in your garden, make sure that it faces north or south since water is the element represented by the northeastern direction.

House Garden Trees and Plants

You can now select the types of trees to plant around your house according to your house direction. Now, before you do that, you must grow your knowledge on which types of trees and plants are the most suitable and highly regarded by Vastu practitioners. Here are the most common trees and plants used in Vastu Shastra practices and where to place them, along with their ideal placements:

Lucky Bamboo Plants

The Lucky Bamboo (scientific name Dracaena braunii) is one of the best plants to have in your garden, as it will attract peace and luck. It should promote health and increase wealth. Be sure not to mistake the Lucky Bamboo with the common bamboo plant, as both vary in shape, size, and effects. Also, avoid the Bonsai and the potted dwarf bamboos, as these are considered going against nature according to Vastu's practices. Lucky Bamboo plants must have a yellow bark instead of a dark-colored one.

Holy Basil Plants

This plant is amongst the best greeneries you can use in your garden. It is highly revered thanks to the positive energy it will bring to your premises. Ideally, it should grow in the north, east, or northeast directions. Also known as Tulsi, the Holy Basil plant is known for bringing auspiciousness and prosperity. As such, it must be used in the right direction to help you reap its benefits.

Flowerpots

While you may be tempted to place flowerpots just about everywhere, flower pots found on the wall, in the east, north, or northeast direction, will effectively block morning sunlight. Even when you feel sunlight coming from these directions, you won't enjoy its full benefits. Instead, you can place flowerpots or any decorative plants on the ground in these directions. Also, remember that they shouldn't grow taller than three feet.

Money Plants

Much like the Lucky Bamboo, the money plant (Epipremnum aureum) is a great source of luck and prosperity. Should you use these plants around your garden, you'll notice a significant increase in your wealth and quality of life. Therefore, you should be mindful of placing these plants to channel their positive effects. For instance, you can place pots of money plants either in the north or east direction, and avoid the south and west orientation.

Ashoka Trees

Ashoka trees, also known as Saraca Indica, should be placed in the south, east, or southeast direction as they are believed to bring joy and mitigate common aches and pain. Planting them in an auspicious direction should magnify these effects. Coconut trees (Cocos nucifera) will have a similar effect, which means you can safely use these trees with the Saraca Indica variety.

Banana Trees

Vastu advocates for planting banana trees in the northeast direction of the house. Also called Musa Genus, these trees enhance physical health and boost mental wellbeing. They also signify peace and serenity. People will even worship this tree, as it is considered sacred.

Mango Trees

Besides their medicinal properties, the leaves of the mango tree are commonly used as pesticides. The twigs can even be used for brushing your teeth. They are highly appreciated from a Vastu viewpoint, so they will be a nice addition to your garden. Plant these trees anywhere but the east or north directions to ward off the adverse and potentially health-damaging effects. Instead, you can plant them in the west direction.

Peonies

Peony flowers are colorful, beautiful, and deeply valued in Vastu practices. They're considered some of the most auspicious flowers and are commonly used in Hindi religious rituals and celebrations. Peonies are also a symbol of feminism and beauty. With their pleasant nature, a lot of Vastu practitioners plant these flowers in their gardens, ideally in the southwest direction.

Plum Blossoms

To invite harmony, wealth, and positive energy into your home, grow plum blossoms (Prunus Mume) in your garden. They're quite eye-pleasing and will promote positive energy all around. These flowers should be placed in the north or northeast direction. But many people believe that their orientation doesn't matter and suggest planting them where you see fit.

Dwarf Jade Plant

Like the spiritual properties of plum blossoms, dwarf jade plants (scientific name Portulacaria Afra) are great sources of positive energy and emit it around the house in abundance. This plant is also believed to attract luck, as it has five leaves, which symbolize the five elements of nature, or "Paanchbhootas." To place these plants in your garden, the north or east direction would be ideal.

Neem Trees

Finally, the Neem tree (Azadirachta Indica) is well known for its medicinal properties and is widely used in traditional holistic healing. Neem trees are also highly regarded in Vastu principles, as they are believed to be one of the most auspicious greeneries in any garden. Many people appreciate the natural flow of air that passes through neem trees directly into their living rooms or bedrooms for therapeutic and a refreshing aroma. Favor placing these trees in a northwest direction.

Roof Gardens and Indoor Plants

The same rules and precepts apply for designing a roof garden. Provided that the plot direction is Vastu-compliant, you can add potted plants and flowers as encouraged by Vastu placement principles. As far as indoor plants, you can use potted Lucky Bamboo plants, money plants, citrus plants, and lavender plants varieties, which will emanate organic, pleasant, and soothing scents in your entire house.

Balconies

Usually Vastu practitioners recommend using small potted plants. Compact and colorful plants should bring plenty of positive energy and allow it to flow about, especially in the right placement. Steer clear of large plants (like creepers) with a tendency to block sunlight effectively, drawing in negative energy and tipping the balance of spiritual influence in your home. Pots will also yield better effects when placed in the west, south, or southwest part of your balcony. Just be sure not to place them at the center to avoid obstructing the flow of energy.

Tips and Tricks

Now that you know more about the varieties of Vast-friendly trees and plants for your home, you're ready to move on to other types of plantations. Your garden can be a collection of shrubs, trees, and flowers that don't aren't mentioned in Vastu teachings. For this, you must know how to place them correctly for them not to interfere with the energy flow and positive effects of other elements in your garden. Here are a couple of useful tips you can follow:

If you're planting shrubs, make sure that they're well placed in the north or east sections of your garden.

Large trees shouldn't be placed too close to your house. The roots of large trees, such as peepal (ficus), can cause irreparable damages to your property. They can also attract rodents, insects, honeybees, etc., which should be avoided since they're considered bad omens.

Tall trees are to be placed in the south, west, and southwest direction of the garden. Likewise, they should also be kept a good distance away from your house to avoid bad luck and negative influences. According to Vastu Shastra principles, their shades should fall on the house between 9 AM and 3 PM.

Avoid thorny plants, like cactus or rose bushes, as they will give off negative energy, which will hinder your garden's positive influences.

Your lawn should be facing north or east. According to Vastu Shastra, a lawn with a swing with a north-south axis will provide multiple opportunities and favorable prospects.

If you're thinking about having a small waterfall installed, it should be placed in the north or east corner directions. Stay clear of the north-east orientation, as misplaced waterfalls or water features can cripple the peace and prosperity of your garden. You may also add a miniature pond with floating lotuses to promote good fortune.

Things to Avoid

There are certain things you must steer clear of to optimize your green space and garner the full benefits of Vastu Shastra. For example, thorny plants, can do more harm than good. They can weaken relationships, increase tension, and trigger fights. Bonsai plants are short, and will encourage stunted growth, either in fortune, career, or relationship matters.

As much as bamboo can be beneficial, it should be kept a fair distance from your house to achieve the best results. Neem trees must also be planted at least 60 meters away from your home. You must avoid adding any item that can inspire tension or violence in your garden, such as a scarecrow, as it will desecrate the peacefulness and serenity you've worked so hard to achieve.

Ultimately, constructing a Vastu-compliant garden can prove a challenging undertaking, especially if you don't have a specific set of instructions or aren't sure of where to start. The best way to tackle this is to take one step at a time, know which direction your home is facing, and then decide which varieties of trees, plants, and flowers you'd like to plant in your garden. It's worth mentioning that, in some scenarios, you might have to remove already-existing elements in your garden to achieve optimum results.

Chapter 9: Pyramids: The Mystery of Energy Concentration

A cornerstone of Vastu Shastra is the pyramid. To understand how it works, one must first go back to Vastu fundamentals. As you now know, Vastu relies on science and the universe's spiritual energy, effectively merging and elevating these two areas of knowledge. Energy channels substance towards the spirit and life, helping them live purposefully and prosperously. Despite being negative this energy creates all that we see in our daily lives and can be centered on the pyramid where it resonates and permeates living beings.

Of Greek origin, the word "pyra" means fire, and "mid" means energy, which explains why the pyramid holds such a strong meaning in Vastu philosophy. The term "pyramid" also denotes a geometrical object which has sides that join at an apex point. Due to the powerful energy that resonates with their unique structures, pyramids are considered powerful objects, which explains why the ancient Egyptians were so keen on using them to build tombs and put life to rest. Energy feeds life into us, and perhaps that was what they were attempting to achieve.

How the Pyramid Works

Typically, there are two rules to how the pyramid works with Vastu Shastra. The one dictates that the energy is highly concentrated around the axis that travels across the pyramid. The second rule holds that the energy is channeled out of the apex of the pyramid. This phenomenon affects all lives and humans and impacts any location's energy levels, helping buildings and homes strike a positive and nurturing balance. This concept is related to bio-geometry, a branch of science that focuses on the study of structures, like pyramids, their dimensions, and their effects on living organisms, particularly humans. For example, conical, square, and pyramidal patterns will all have various bearings on human bodies or living organisms. Incidentally, how energy is channeled in Vastu Shastra differs from how it is used in Feng Shui, as both have their own approaches and methods for funneling energies.

How They Can Be Used

In Vastu, the pyramid can be a pivotal center of energy in your house and possibly your entire existence. Therefore, countless people use it for blocking negative energy and drawing in the more positive influences. To unlock the secrets of this iconic instrument for your home, here are several useful pointers:

Thanks to their effectiveness in dispelling negative energies, Vastu pyramids are used in homes, especially at the corner of the house, for an optimal effect.

If you have an impaired energy flow in a certain room, you can reenergize that space by adding Vastu pyramids to all four corners. Once you're done with that step, you'll notice a sense of coordination and positivity taking effect in the room.

If you're concerned about energy levels in the workspace, particularly in your office, you can place one pyramid on your desk. Aside from acting as a nice décor item, you'll soon notice a more positive and conducive ambiance.

Due to their ability to channel large quantities of energy in any space, you can carry on with your meditative practices under one pyramid. This should help strengthen your mental faculties, concentration, and boost your meditation experience at once.

Vastu pyramids can also be kept underwater to support the positive energy flow across your metabolic water balance. If you experience digestion issues or stomach aches, placing Vastu pyramids underwater will help you.

Like the above, the Vastu pyramid can preserve your food items or any products you possess for a substantial amount of time.

Placement

Following the placement and directions of Vastu guides can appear a daunting task, especially for novices. Luckily, the Vastu pyramid placement isn't as difficult as following other, more complex Vastu precepts. They can either be placed in a central point, at the corners, or any location in which energy is most prominent. You can also place them in your bedroom, office, car, or simply even in your pocket.

The Various Types of the Vastu Pyramid

While they essentially share the same shape, Vastu pyramids can vary in quality, material, and size. You have the liberty to choose whichever type of Vastu pyramid appeals to you the most, as they will all serve the purpose of purifying and concentrating positive energy in your surroundings. However, it never hurts to learn more about the Vastu pyramid's different iterations, along with their unique characteristics and properties.

Promax Pyramids

These pyramids are known for their power to produce large quantities of energies through their nine-layer energy grid. The Promax top and gold plate are located at the sides and both channel energy; they are supported by an energy plate at the bottom of the pyramid. They're generally used when working on the land, building construction, financial and investment operations, and miscellaneous projects. So, use this pyramid on these premises.

Flat Max Pyramids

As the name suggests, these pyramids are flat and are specifically designed for apartments. By using one pyramid in your flat, it'll help you magnify energy concentrations, which will instantly increase the flow of positive energies and boost your home's spiritual value. This may include better energy balance, wealth, and a more prosperous lifestyle. You can also use these pyramids in shops, factories, or large family homes.

Agro Pyramid

If you're struggling to grow your garden, agro pyramids will be the most suitable solution in this scenario. Agro pyramids foster an immense, mystical power that can influence the growth and distribution of good grain with little effort. They should also improve the quality of your greenery, vegetables, fruits, and herbs, so you can use them in your garden for that purpose.

Super Max Pyramids

As mentioned earlier, pyramids will have similar effects in cleansing your location of negative energies and concentrating on the positive ones. In that regard, many Vastu practitioners claim that supermax pyramids will have an even greater magnifying effect. They're ideal in situations where the energy balance is leaning towards the negative side. These pyramids usually have a gold center, which explains why you're bound to experience an exponential increase in energy. These can be used anywhere, but they're more prevalent in homes and offices. Supermax pyramids can also increase your wealth and health, so they're one of the best Vastu pyramids you can decorate your space with.

Multi-Tier 9 x 9 Pyramid

The multi-tier 9 x 9 pyramid is known for its Vastu and Feng Shui curative properties. It's mostly used in Vastu remedies to optimize energy balance and is also capable of land charging and activating the room's center. Most of the multi-tier 9 x 9 pyramids contain neutron polymers to achieve effective and immediate results once the pyramid is used. It's also made up of a pyra top, a pyra plate, and nine pyra chips, which are fixed to the base of the pyramid with adhesive material. Depending on your needs and the space's configuration, you can place that pyramid on the ground, on a desk, attach it to your ceiling, or fix it to a wall.

Bemor 9 x 9 Pyramid

If you're looking for a Vastu-approved apparatus to enhance your luck (aside from arranging your house according to the favored direction), Bemor 9 x 9 pyramids should be your go-to choice. These pyramids improve their users' luck and energize their homes, much like the other pyramids listed here. These pyramids will often be found around office spaces, where they can increase wealth and income, and homes to attract and hoard the much-needed positive energy. Bemor pyramids come with nine pyra chips, one pyra plate, and a lotus power hole plate.

Which Material to Opt For

As you may already know, the first built pyramids were made from rock stones, but now, there are several options you can choose from, from rare metals to ordinary plastic. Before you decide which material to select, you must decide the purpose of the activity you'll be using the pyramid for. For instance, if you will use it for yoga, concentration, or any meditative activity, your ideal choice will be stone. But plastic or glass pyramids are better suited for energy magnification, yet must be kept in bright, well-lit locations.

In parallel, crystal pyramids won't only embrace the positive energy, but they'll also prevent negativity from entering your house. Pyramids made of this precious material are also ideal for healing sickness, improving mental faculties, enhancing your intuition, and even losing weight. This will depend on the crystal you're using, though. For example, agate will have a significant calming effect. Bloodstone will promote good blood circulation and cardiovascular health. Moonstone is more appropriate for the ladies, as it works on improving feminine health. Clear quartz is ideal for meditative activities. Finally, snowflake obsidian will help boost your immune system. If you will use crystal pyramids, make sure that you have four to be placed at each corner of the room to reap maximum benefits.

Benefits of Vastu Pyramids

By now, you may have guessed that the main purpose of Vastu pyramids is to direct positive energy towards you and your house. However, the benefits you will garner from these powerful items will build up eventually. After a few months of using Vastu pyramids, you'll notice tremendous changes in your life. The following outlines the changes you'll most likely experience.

Wealth and Prosperity

According to Vastu precepts, the idea according to which money can't buy happiness is null. Vastu Shastra acknowledges that it can indeed affect our lives. This is why most of Vastu's practices harness cosmic energy to bring wealth and financial prosperity to their users. Within months of using Vastu pyramids, be it in your office or at your house, you'll notice that both your fortune and income will have increased, which will help you enjoy a better lifestyle for both you and your family.

Love Life

Many people struggle with their personal relationships for years on end. Some will even think that they'll never meet their soulmate or find true love. Using Vastu pyramids can alter your perspective. Once the right placement of the pyramids is achieved, positive energies will attract a potential companion who brings happiness and harmony into your life. If marriage is your goal, then you're bound to have a happy and long-lasting one when using a Vastu pyramid.

Family

Vastu pyramids can affect our relationships with our entourage. To build a loving, harmonious family, adding the right Vastu pyramids to your home will get you closer to that aspiration. Remember, though, that you should at least be familiar with Vastu practices for this to work. As discussed in the previous chapter, thorny plants in your garden (cactus, roses) can interfere with the energies emitted by the pyramids, hence the importance of strategic placement. Family plays a central role in our lives, so you must follow Vastu's recommendations to the letter to nurture peaceful and cordial relationships with your loved ones.

Health

Invariably, pyramids are most often used to improve one's health. Few things can stop you from making progress as much as impaired health, be it in your work, relationships, or your meditation goals. Pyramids work to negative energies and their damaging effects. By using the right type and number of pyramids, you'll be able to maintain a disease-free environment and protect your home's occupants from illness and health-related conditions.

Education

Education is a quintessential aspect of your children's lives. To see your children grow to their fullest potential, you must give them the best education you can afford as any caring parent would. While Vastu pyramids won't have a direct hand in this, they can always bring your children positive and rewarding opportunities for their development. They'll improve their cognitive functions, concentration, and overall health, all of which will promise them to stellar education and career.

Protection and Purification

As established, one objective of Vastu Shastra is to dispel any evil or negative energy from your living and working environment. Pyramids can serve as a potent source of protection against this devilry. They should also take instant effect once you place them correctly around your space. You can also place Vastu pyramids in your car to make sure your safety and that of all passengers.

Other Vastu Tools

While diverting your interest in Vastu pyramids, you mustn't neglect to combine them with other tools to optimize the pooling of positive energies in your home. For instance, Vastu sleep is a useful tool you can keep under your mattress. Its purpose is to garner the benefits of cosmic energies and improve the quality of your sleep. If your mind is often troubled, and you find yourself prone to chronic insomnia, you can use Vastu sleep to soothe your body, spirit, and mind. It should also work in harmony with pyramids placed in your bedroom to foster success, enhance your health, and promote serenity.

Another instrument you can use with the pyramids is the pyra cap. Pyra caps are basically pyramid-shaped accessories you can wear on your head during your meditation sessions. They're said to improve mind power during meditation, especially when the practice is conducted under a pyramid. Acquiring a pyra cap is a must if you're channeling Vastu Shastra for meditation or yoga. Pyra caps improve concentration and confidence. They can also help your mind relax and alleviate stress without you having to take any medication. To reap the full benefits of a meditation session, you should use a pyra cap.

Pyramid Roof

While pyramid roofs are not technically considered Vastu pyramids, people have reported these roofs carry surprising effectiveness. It's also recommended that you create a pyramid roof for your living room if it's the central part of your house, which it generally is. Sitting under a pyramid roof will positively influence your memory power, reduce backaches, headaches, and be a remedy to your insomnia. If you're going to place pyramids in other parts of your house, make sure that one of the triangles faces north.

This should also be the case for your pyramid roof; in fact, pyramid roofs can have an even more powerful effect than small-sized pyramids and will work in harmony with other pyramidal structures placed in the corners of your house.

All in all, Vastu pyramids are essential for any Vastu practitioner. Given how easy it is to use them, you won't have to deal with the confusion of directions and orientations often associated with Vastu. Fortunately, these pyramids come in all shapes and sizes, and each type boasts its own unique properties and set of benefits. To ensure you get the best Vastu pyramid for your house or workspace, you must document yourself further to decide which one would be ideal according to your needs and aspirations. The energy that comes from these pyramids is primordial for humans, living beings, and our planet, so it's only fair it must be channeled correctly and purified from any negative, potentially noxious influences.

Chapter 10: Destructive Vastu Remedies

The ideal way to build a home or a workplace that abides by the majority of Vastu principles is by making sure that they're implemented right from the beginning of the conception and building phase. Now, since not many people know the Vastu concepts or aren't convinced of their effects and benefits early on, this aspect is largely overlooked. Fortunately, it's possible to instill the right energy and frequency, even if your home or workplace wasn't built according to the precepts of Vastu Shastra. While this chapter's name has nothing to do with actual destruction or ruin, it is rather about rebuilding and renovation to resolve a challenging situation through the effective use and implementation of Vastu principles.

Considerations Before Applying the Principles

When you start putting what you've learned from Vastu Shastra into practice, you'll notice that it can be quite flexible. There are no hard or rigid rules that will prevent you from inviting harmony and prosperity into your home or workplace the way you see it. Vastu science sees a building or space as a living organism, making it possible to approach it from different perspectives. Achieving even half of the principles of Vastu is considered a job well done. It's important to perceive the space that you're trying to build or decorate as an integral part of yourself, intact with your frequency and vibrations. By respecting the laws of nature, you're ensuring that the space is harmoniously balanced, which is why it shouldn't be tackled as yet another tedious renovation job.

One of the most important considerations to factor into this process is the individuals' unique characteristics and personalities in a workspace or home. You shouldn't think of the space as your own because if other people spend a lot of time in it, their thoughts and needs are bound to be an element of consideration in any Vastu remedy. Think of your space as a temple that deeply nurtures your spirit and soul; building it properly becomes primordial to make sure that your spirituality and internal energy balance are prosperous and well-guarded.

No matter how one tries to put it, the physical space you spend most of your time in will necessarily affect you in a variety of ways, for better or worse. This is why Vastu principles are highly sought after, namely, to ensure that the effects always tip towards the positive side. You may need to take a moment to analyze yourself, your lifestyle, and your needs, to discover a pattern that can make sure your personal comfort and convenience.

Proceeding with Care

When you use destructive Vastu remedies, it's always important to be careful about the changes you're planning. As explained, buildings and their surroundings should be treated as organisms that foster fluctuating energies. Modifying a space too much and in the wrong direction can hinder the vibrations and energy of the place, ultimately disrupting your own harmony and spiritual balance. It's best to draw a design copy of the alterations you want to make and use a Vastu blueprint that incorporates the five elements to tell whether your modifications would be harming any of them, albeit slightly. Fire and water elements are often the most clashing elements in many setups, especially those in the kitchen (faucets, ovens, etc.).

Invariably, there are several drawbacks to a kitchen that doesn't follow The Vastu principles. If you enjoy cooking and spending a lot of time in your home kitchen, you might be putting a lot at stake if you choose not to follow the Vastu guidelines. Chronic conditions and inexplicable diseases can affect the house chef if the cooking space is teeming with malicious vibrations caused by inauspicious furniture and hardware placement, along with an inadequate orientation of the kitchen. There is also the possibility of arising family problems, which can upset even the strongest of relationships.

How to Redesign your Kitchen

Since the kitchen is one of the core areas of any house, using destructive Vastu remedies can effectively help cleanse it of any bad energy.

The Placement of the Space

If you're still deciding where to place the kitchen, it's recommended to go for the southeast direction, where the fire element is dominant. If that's not feasible, you can also choose a northwest orientation.

Placement of Stove and Sink

Align your stove in the southeast direction to establish that the person using it is always facing east. In parallel, make sure that the sinks and taps are placed on the opposite side of the stove, as water and fire elements should never mingle. The flowing of the water should abide by a northeast direction to promote positive and rewarding energies.

Placement of the Refrigerator

Try to find a location for the refrigerator that isn't in the northeast direction. Avoid placing it in a corner. Generally, you should place no electrical appliances in the northeast direction of the kitchen.

Placement of Storage and Water Vessels

You can choose either the western or eastern side of your space for storage. For the water vessels, you'll want to go toward water, which should be on the northeastern side of your kitchen.

Design and Colors

Suppose you're in the right state of energy to renovate your kitchen and make it Vastu-compliant. In that case, favor ceramic tiles or marble material for the floorings because of their durability and consistency. Adding a few colors may be overlooked by many people, but this is an essential element in any space's energy optimization process. In the southeast corner of your kitchen, try adding hues of soft red. If you're handling the kitchen flooring, best to go with white, off-white, creamy, or light gray colors to give it a solid look and grounded feel. Also, please go for expressive colors like red, yellow, orange, or purple for the décor. You can rarely go wrong with most colors in the kitchen, to the exception of black, which you should avoid because of the negative energy it can harbor.

Leveraging Vastu to Prevent Theft

One of Vastu designs' many benefits is its proven effect in controlling external factors that can hinder your well-being. Theft is one of the most common ailments that can plague a non-Vastu-compliant home. This doesn't mean that Vastu will prevent all types of theft as if it were a steel gate, but it can keep a lot of problems at bay when you address it early on. The location of the door, its direction, the material it's made of, and many factors are features in the Vastu practice to help avert the incidence of thefts.

If you own valuables like jewelry or cash that you'd like to keep in the house, avoid placing it on the northwest side since it can increase instructions and break-ins.

Always make sure that the main entrance to your home is noticeably bigger than any other door in your house.

If you have multiple doors and windows, make sure that their number is an even number.

Use sacred symbols as decorations beside the entrance doors.

Obstructions to the house's main entrance should be removed because they disrupt the energy flow both inside and outside the house.

Avoid photographs, posters, or art that portray a malicious or evil aura (scenes of horror, violence, or despair) as this can bring in noxious energies.

Understanding the Necessity of Demolitions

Many people are reluctant to destroying a piece of their property, even when they know it can be for the best. Most Vastu consultants will try their best to work out a way to avoid demolition, but when that's inexorable, some extra work is due. One dilemma you might face, for example, is a toilet or staircase in the northeast direction. While Feng Shui may offer solutions to alleviate the negative energy through certain items, it won't be more than a temporary solution; removing these structures is sometimes the only remedy.

If you plan on applying Vastu principles to the letter, you must let go of any reluctance you may have about destructive remedies. If a structure is causing a clash with Vastu tenets in the house, you must remove it. Not that it's the only way, but you need to be mentally prepared for worst-case scenarios.

Dealing with Wells and Extensions

If you live in a house with a well in the property's southeast direction, you might need to remove it or bury it with mud or stone. Many people use lids to close the wells, but this isn't the most effective way. Permanent solutions are the best way to deal with these structures to avoid future, potentially costly hassles.

Extensions leaning towards the northwest section in a property are notoriously difficult to resolve without using destructive Vastu remedies. You can start by adjusting the boundaries of that extension or implementing a doorway to delimit a northeastern corner to mitigate that direction's effect. You may be tempted to place idols instead of doing this, but that will only temporarily solve a part of the problem.

Painting the Walls

Depending on the state of your interior walls, a paint job can be considered both a destructive and non-destructive Vastu remedy. You cannot randomly paint the walls hoping for harmonious results. You need to consider the room you are painting to ensure compliance with the Vastu principles.

Living Room

The living room is a very important section of your house and is usually the first your visitors are introduced to. As such, you'll want to make it look bold and lively by using warm and energetic colors like blue, yellow, off-white, and green. Add a hint of red for an added energy boost, but in moderation.

Dining Room

The dining room's colors should reflect good health and prosperity, so choosing relaxing colors that can put you in a state of ease is highly recommended. Blue, pink, and green are all viable options you can paint the walls with for the most tranquil and soothing effect.

Master Bedroom

The bedroom should always induce a sense of relaxation, besides little hints of romantic vitality. The most favored colors are blue, pink, or purple. Avoid darker shades of these colors to maintain a tranquil and effective color scheme.

Guest Bedroom

The guest bedroom is generally designed for temporary stays, which means you can offer more than the usual relaxing colors by choosing light shades of yellow, orange, or lavender. These colors can exude a royal sense of belonging and intimacy to your visiting guests.

Study or Work Room

For this space, you'll want to select colors that promote concentration, and according to Vastu, those would be green, blue, and purple in their lightest shades to avoid distractions and loss of focus. This should help make the environment comfortable and pleasant enough to boost your productivity and mental faculties.

Bathroom

People always consider their bathroom to be the most private and even the safest space around their homes. It should always give off relaxing vibrations. The colors you should use for these rooms should be dark shades of black, gray, white, pink, or a mix of them all. Elegance and comfort should be combined to secure that your bathroom is aesthetically pleasing and conducive to a good energy balance.

Renovations in the Bedroom

Whatever you're trying to achieve, avoid having a bedroom in the southeast direction. According to the most basic Vastu precepts, these rooms should be in almost any corner except the southeastern one. If you already have a bedroom in there, relocate it all together. As a temporary solution, you can shift the bed away from the room's corner to avoid the fire vibrations in this quadrant. If you have a master bedroom with an adjacent bathroom, you'll want to make sure it's directed towards the east or north sides of the room. It's also essential to keep the attached bathroom door always closed, and to keep the toilet seat down. Because of Vastu principles, mirrors shouldn't be in the bedroom if you have a partner because they can lead to frequent fights and tense up the environment. However, if you find that a mirror is an essential item in your bedroom, then try to place it on the northeastern wall of the room.

Renovations in the Living Room

The living room is the heart of your house and its influence extends well beyond the walls that bind it. This signifies that having negative vibrations in the living room can resonate in other rooms as well. Idols, paintings, and other decorations are great additions, but they shouldn't be your main point of focus unless you make sure that the living room is properly Vastu-compliant first. Here are useful living room arrangement and renovations tips:

You can choose between the northwest, northeast, northern, and southwest directions if you're planning to move your living room. The perfect setup for those who don't like parties or having company over is usually the northwestern section of your house, as it belongs to the air quadrant, which depicts activity and movement. The southwestern location is ideal for get-togethers and late-night parties because visitors always prefer this direction. If you're looking to foster positive energy coupled with nature's calm tranquility, the northeastern location is a sure-fire option.

Assess if you can restructure the beams or girders on the ceiling because they can induce stress, a sense of heaviness, and inauspicious vibes.

If the living room entrance is in the southwestern corner, you might need to restructure the entrance to move it toward the western direction.

Vastu in the Office

If you're managing an office you must attend to countless details that can cause a myriad of issues if left unchecked. If your office is facing east, try shifting the balance towards the west because it brings strength, stability, and balance. Try to remove any office-related equipment from the northeastern section of the space and move the water resources over there. You may also need to relocate the staircase if it stands in the center of the office because it can disrupt energy flow. The reception should almost always be in the northeastern direction, which can be problematic if the staircase is in the space.

The majority of destructive Vastu remedies shouldn't be attempted solo if you have no experience in renovations or DIY projects. Your best bet is to solicit the services of a professional Vastu consultant to help guide you through the process, no matter how much work is required. Ultimately, tackling these issues is primordial if you're planning on transforming your house or office into a Vastu-compliant paradise.

Chapter 11: Non-Destructive Vastu Remedies

Understanding the science of Vastu Shastra enables you to eradicate any source of harmful energy in your building. Learning more about the balance and dynamics of energy gives you a chance to harness positive ones for your gains without having to destroy or demolish your surroundings. While the science of Vastu might revolve around directions, cosmic energies need to be considered as well. The energy emitted by your belongings (property, furniture, décor items) should not be neglected throughout your journey. Think of Vastu as a balance you can bring to your home or workspace with non-destructive remedies. The majority of Vastu experts believe that mental and physical impairments, mostly, result from ignoring Vastu principles. Neglecting the application of Vastu remedies in your living space can lead to financial issues, given how difficult it will be to contribute your best work. To help you in repelling bad energies and welcoming good vibes in your building, this chapter will delve into the characteristics and applications of non-destructive Vastu remedies.

Walls and Colors

In Vastu, walls are considered the foundation of any building; they represent support and strength. This is the first element to consider when you're trying to balance energies and fill your house with positivity. Since colors hold a lot of weight, they require proper attention and care. Even if you live in an already-finished home, it's easy to repaint the walls to foster good energy and prosperity. Color theory isn't just about matching colors on a wheel, but, it's a science you must delve into to select the right colors for the energies you wish to attract. Invariably, the aesthetic and palette you choose should align with your inner self; neglecting this aspect might make you feel out of place and detached from the place. It's imperative to consider Vastu principles and the color theory and choose the colors you feel connected with the most.

Warm, strong colors such as red represent passion, vibrancy, and liveliness. Given these attributes, you must be cautious with it. For example, your bedroom should never be painted in red because this will promote discomfort and make you angry and on edge. But red works great in living rooms as it suggests warmth and high energy. Yellow is another warm color that signifies boldness and courage. It emits feelings of warmth, elation, and optimism. While yellow is best used combined with other colors to elevate a room and make it appear larger, it's suitable for children's bedrooms. However, choose lighter or more faded shades of the color, like soft pastels.

Cold colors such as blue or green are more calming, soothing, and grounding. It's no wonder why blue has been regarded as the color of eternal beauty across time and cultures. It's the color of the sky and the sea that evokes tranquility and serenity. According to Vastu precepts, blue is more suited for large areas where you need peace and calmness. In parallel, green is one of the best cold colors for attracting wealth, stability, and promoting individual growth. When you repaint a wall in lime, sage, mint, or sea-foam, it changes the mood of the room and makes space become more soothing and welcoming.

Lighting

The late Martin Luther King Jr. famously once said that darkness could not drive out darkness; only light can do so. This quote is inspired by Hindu philosophy and its interest in studying different light sources, along with how the impact of their placement. Harnessing positive energies in your living or working space cannot be achieved without the right lighting. Let's explore how lighting can do wonders for your space with just a few simple changes:

Never ignore filling your space with good lighting; light can effectively transform any room's feel and atmosphere. Good lighting can have a positive, uplifting effect on your mood and mental state. So, always start by allowing a source of bright light, especially around your house's main door, to attract positivity and prosperity.

Make sure that the corners of every room are well lit. Not only will this illuminate your space and make it seem wider and more pleasant to the eye, but it also welcomes good vibes into your space.

Natural sunlight is key to balancing energies in your house, hence the importance of ensuring that your whole building, especially your home office or workplace, has constant access to natural light. This will provide warmth and stability to your space while bringing in vibes of joy and comfort that will boost your productivity and concentration.

The light emanating from fireplaces and candles is naturally soothing and relaxing and usually fit best in the living room, bathroom, and bedroom. This will elevate the mood of these rooms to transform them into peaceful and relaxing dens.

In Hindu philosophy, it's believed that the northeastern corner of any space is the Sattva corner, which represents one of the three essential modes of existence. The majority of Vastu experts also believe that allowing natural light to enter from this corner symbolizes creativity, positive energy, and wealth for the occupants. Negativity, on the other hand, is represented by the southwestern corner. As such, you must make sure that the main sources of lighting in any space is placed in the sattva corner.

Finally, your bathroom lighting shouldn't be overlooked, especially the ones surrounding the mirror. The light you need to add to this area should be diffused and not display any glares or shadows.

Vastu For Bedrooms

Many people don't find comfort in their own bedrooms when this should be their space for comfort and relaxation, which is always a demoralizing prospect. Without comfort in your bedroom, you'll be more likely to feel worn out and stressed. Applying the Vastu principles can prove highly beneficial for optimizing and harmonizing your bedroom for an unparalleled living and resting experience. Consider these useful pointers:

According to ancient Vastu beliefs, the southwest corner of the building is the ideal location for the bedroom as it's believed to attract longevity, health, and prosperity.

The northwest corner is more suitable for children or guest bedrooms. The northeast and southeast corners should be avoided as they're believed to increase physical health issues, mental health challenges, and household conflicts.

If you live in a house that already has bedrooms in its northeast or southeast corners, there are some non-destructive remedies to balance out the negative energies. For instance, you may use lavender essential oil or incense sticks to compensate for any structural defects your house might have. Another remedy you can safely use involves placing small bowls of coarse or sea salt in each corner of the room to fill it with good energy and repel any negative ones.

As per the Vastu tradition, your bed should ideally be placed in the southwest corner of the room. When sleeping, make sure that your head points to either the south or the east. Otherwise, this will prevent your body from absorbing positive and rejuvenating vibrations. But it's been established that a couple sharing a bed should always sleep with their heads towards the south and their legs pointing to the north.

Vastu principles dictate that the shape of your bed should be a rectangle or a square. Generally, it is best to steer clear of unconventional shapes for furniture pieces around the home. The most suitable material for your bed is wood, ideally the organic, non-recycled kind.

According to Vastu specialists, placing the bed under a beam or near a sidewall is a big no-no. However, you could always have a fake ceiling installed to avoid this common oversight. Also, make sure that there's enough room around it for you to access the bed easily from both sides.

Artwork and Plants

Paintings, artwork, and interior plants are an integral part of any culture and design philosophy. But people are questioning their painting choices, for foregoing artworks altogether for fear of selecting illustrations that might attract negative energies or evil forces. This habit stems from the confusion that many people experience when trying to choose pictures compliant with Vastu to complement their houses. Invariably, artwork and house plants are excellent choices for houses and buildings to promote growth and happy vibes and make the space beautiful and well put together. Here are a few tips to aid you in your search for auspicious decorative items that will bring your home together in harmony and unity.

If your living room has a southwest wall, make use of it to hang a family portrait with a bright spotlight that highlights the photo. This is believed to bring health, luck, and good fortune for the family members.

Avoid representations of violence, suffering, or death in your artwork. Instead, choose inspiring and visually pleasing subjects such as natural landscapes, exotic destinations, geometric patterns, or whatever strikes your fancy.

To harness positive energies and trap them into your house, bamboo plants will be your go-to for good luck. The most popular choice nowadays is the money plant, yet you need to be careful about its placement. As explained in a previous chapter, it should be placed in the southern or northern corner of the room to attract wealth and fortune. With plants, you can get creative if you choose positive colors you feel connected to. You can arrange different colorful flowers and plants such as purple orchids or plum blossoms that suggest positivity and wealth.

Some plants don't have a place inside in the house, including thorny plants like cacti because they're believed to attract negative energies and inauspiciousness. Also avoid plants that hamper growth, such as miniature bonsai trees. If you're a fan of big plants, best to avoid placing them in the northern corner of your space as they might hinder positive vibes.

Vastu-compliant decorative items aren't simply limited to paintings and plants. For example, adding a crystal chandelier to your living room can effectively attract good tidings to your space. However, balance it out with the other elements. You can also make use of candles with artful holders to impart aesthetics, warmth, and contentment in your living area.

Mirrors

Adding the right mirrors in terms of shape, placement, and size can be tricky to master. Adding mirrors plays a huge role in reflecting your whole house with positive vibes and expelling negative energy. Mirrors are also considered a quick fix for the removal of Vastu-related troubles. According to Vastu Shastra, there are three fundamental rules to observe for optimal mirror placement. The first rule is to never place a mirror facing the main door as it's said to harbor inauspiciousness and cause turbulence in the home. The second guideline dictates you shouldn't put up a mirror that directly faces your bed, as it can be a great source of harm and instability in the household. Finally, placing two mirrors in front of each other should also be avoided to prevent magnifying any bad energy that might be lurking around your space.

With a few simple tricks, you can attend to any Vastu shortcomings your house might be enduring. When applying these principles, the most important thing is to choose what best suits your personality and energy profile. When focusing on making your home Vastu-friendly, always be sure to select designs and dispositions that reflect your preferences. This will help you optimize the space in a unique, effortless, and harmonious fashion.

Chapter 12: Feng Shui Remedies for Harmonious Living

As we've learned early on, the term Feng Shui literally translates to "wind-water" and signifies a harmonious flow of energy. Feng Shui works in such a way that it's made many people believe it's a form of magic reserved for a privileged few with strong intuitive psychic powers. In reality, Feng Shui is merely but a philosophical system with well-defined rules and beliefs that can effectively transform any dwelling into a harmonious and united space filled with positive energy. Feng Shui is considered a science that takes both the Earth's and cosmic energies into account. While it might seem a complex and esoteric concept, much like Vastu Shastra, the trick is to avoid jumping right into its precepts without a proper understanding of its benefits and applications. You can start with simple yet effective remedies to turn your space into a healthy and harmonious environment that reflects positively on you and your family's mental state, physical health, and achievements in life. Let's see how you can achieve this delicate balance with ease.

Perfect Your Center Point

As with any design philosophy, it's crucial to pay attention to every detail that goes into forming your living space. According to Feng Shui's principles, the center of your living space harbors the utmost gravity. This essentially means that, to balance out the different energies to achieve harmony, stability, and contentment, you must make sure that the heart of your home fosters spiritual nourishment and positive energy. The house's center is usually called the *Yin-Yang point*, where all opposites meet and blend with one another. This elemental point should look pleasing, feel comfortable, and have a coherent design to bring balance and harmony to your space. You may also place your favorite décor items at the center of your house to allow your spirit and soul to be surrounded by peace, beauty, and harmoniousness.

Aim for a More Welcoming Entry Path

Chi refers to the balance between Yin and Yang; it's the energy of life and the center around which the universe revolves. In Feng Shui, your home's exterior entrance leading to the main door is believed to be the opening of Chi. This is a gateway for positive energies that support growth, wealth, and fortune. As such, it's imperative to embellish your entry path by filling it with greenery and beautiful, soothing lights. You can also go the extra mile by adding an assortment of fragrant, dopamine-stimulating flowers. Likewise, add anything that makes you feel more energized, happy, and comforted, such as a collection of crystals, stress-relieving objects, small water fountains, illustrations, or chimes. Another thing to consider, according to Feng Shui, is that you and your family should make it a habit to always use your house's front door as the main entry gate. Using the back door can pave the way for negative and harmful energies to permeate your home.

Always Declutter

Cluttered spaces are often considered the root of all evil, especially in rooms where you're meant to be relaxing or getting work done. You can dedicate a few hours of your time every week to look around the house for anything you no longer have a use for, from shrunken clothes to worn-out furniture pieces and dysfunctional appliances. So, get rid of these items regularly to avoid pile-ups and non-optimal exploitation of your surface area. Cluttered spaces affect us on different levels consciously and subconsciously as they can increase stress levels and hinder wellbeing and productivity. It's also believed that a messy home promotes a wish to add more to your possessions until you end up becoming a compulsive hoarder. But material objects can never offer that level of satisfaction and fulfillment that most of us expect from buying clothes, electronics, and all those things that litter our interiors pointlessly.

Functionality is Essential

While the science and practice of Feng Shui are typically associated with spirituality and energy balance, there exists an indirect link between the flow of energy and the functionality of the objects found in any home. Postponing minor repairs or replacements might hamper the natural flow of Chi and make way for negative energies to proliferate in your space. You must always ensure that everything in your house is in order and functioning as it should. Fix jammed doors, change light bulbs, repair broken fans or air conditioning vents, attend to leaks, and even change batteries yourself if you can. Where possible, always mend the flaws yourself unless it's something you genuinely cannot do, such as HVAC, advanced electrics, plumbing, etc.

Leave Work Out of the Bedroom

In today's world, many people have resorted to remote or freelance work, either by choice or due to global circumstances. This has led many to develop the habit of working in bed or from their bedrooms' comfort. According to Feng Shui precepts, this is a big no-no. The bedroom should serve its purpose relaxation only, sleeping, and enjoyment. You should never invite energies of stress, impatience, and restlessness into your bedroom by turning it into a workstation. If you're working from home, dedicate a space in your living room or an entire room to turn into a work corner or home office. This will help establish healthy boundaries in your interior, which will bring stability and optimize all its occupants' wellbeing.

Harmonious Bedroom

Now that we've established one of the cardinal rules about the bedroom, the following helpful bedroom tips will promote harmony and unity within your sacred space:

Start by placing your bed in such a way it has a solid wall behind it. By doing this, you'll bring energies of stability and comfort your way. This is essential for proper, quality sleep. Applying this simple change will help you rest and recuperate faster and better, which works to boost your productivity and concentration levels during the daytime.

Just like in Vastu Shastra, there should be enough room on both sides of the bed. Also, avoid placing your bed under a beam as it can inhibit the flow of positive energy. This oversight can lead to chronic stress and mental impairments because your room's energy is pressured under the beam.

Make it a habit to open your bedroom door and any windows for at least half an hour each day. This will allow fresh energy to flow into your room. Replenishing the Chi energy in your bedroom helps bring good fortune and prosperity, aside from necessary ventilation and ambient air renewal.

In the art of Feng Shui, mirrors can be the perfect tool for bringing positive vibes and desirable energies, placed the mirror is optimal. For example, placing any mirrors in the opposite direction of the bed is a big no-no, as it's said to bring a third party in the relationship and increase marital conflicts.

Your bedroom should only satisfy its purpose and be conducive to relaxation and good health. Aside from work and ill-placed mirrors, having a television in the bedroom is also advised against. If you cannot get rid of this habit, though, then the next best thing is to cover up the TV screen when not in use or choose an installation that can conceal the TV behind a mobile wall.

Understand the Energy Map

To achieve harmony and fill your space with happiness, relaxation, and unity using the precepts of Feng Shui, you need to understand the eight essential areas connected to several aspects of your life. This is called using compass readings of Bagua to define the different areas in your space. Starting with the north, which represents career and life path and is related to blue and the water element of Feng Shui. But the south portrays the fire element and is linked to warm, vibrant colors such as red, pink, orange, and yellow. The south suggests fame and reputation; it's the light you carry inside you that helps you learn your identity and values. This direction also reflects the perception other people have of you. Since water is almost always associated with blue and black, avoid using these colors in the southern corner of your house for elemental balance.

Symbolized by the colors green and brown, which are linked to the wood element, the east relates to a house's residents' health. Using these colors in the eastern corner will improve health and balance the family vibes inside the household. In the west, best to use white shades to foster creativity and fertility energy. Other areas are represented by the five elements, which are wood, fire, earth, metal, and water. While they're linked to different colors and shapes, learning how to follow this energy map accurately will reflect positively on various aspects of your life, including physical health, mental wellness, and success in your professional life.

Use the Northern Corner of the House Strategically

Since the northern corner of the house suggests your career and life paths according to Feng Shui, you should make the most of it. The northern element is water and is represented by different shades of blue and black. Placing a body of water, such as a fountain or a fish tank, is the ideal way to garner all the positive and nourishing energies that will propel you forward, whether in your personal, social, or professional life. Placing any water body in this corner of a building is proven to induce marked improvements in health, wealth, happiness, and soaking family members with auras of positivity and harmony. An aquarium attracts fortune and financial prosperity; however, one must be careful to not botch it as this could lead to loss of income, bankruptcy, possible lawsuits, and a host of negative repercussions.

Beware of The Poison Arrows

In Feng Shui, it's believed that any sharp or pointed objects naturally channel negative energies. They can wreak havoc on your house by spoiling its balance and harmony. To prevent this from happening, avoid having any pointed objects such as sharp corners, roof angles, buildings with pointed ends, or overhead beams that might foster noxious energies, bring bad luck, impact health, cause missed opportunities, and more. Such sharp objects are often called *poison arrows* or "*the killing breath*," a fitting term for the concept.

Do Not Disturb the Flow

The energy of Feng Shui is positive, smooth, and flows. In that optic, it's essential to make sure that your house harbors no objects that might disrupt the flux of positive energies. This is why best to do away with decorative items that might be too gaudy or ostentatious and disrupt this flow. This is up to preferences. If you're a fan of paintings and artwork, adorning your space with the right pieces in the right places will help in achieving a more harmonious space. If you find that some art pieces, light fixtures, or any décor items are distracting then best to get rid of them. Don't be tempted to hang on to possessions that might push negative energies your way.

The art of Feng Shui can feel intricate, to some extent. When you're first stepping foot on this territory, it's recommended to start with the simple and easy-to-implement home arrangement and decoration tips. As you'll have noted, the aforementioned suggestions require no destruction or demolishing. You can simply start by paying attention to the five essential elements, the colors associated with them, and their overall balance to effectively transform your space into a more welcoming, harmonious environment that will foster prosperity and auspiciousness inside your household.

Conclusion

Congratulations on reaching the end of this book! The chapters gave you a comprehensive overview, so you don't feel the need to move between the chapters should you be searching for something in particular. It's always recommended to read more on the history of Vastu Shastra and Feng Shui to understand the context of these last few chapters. Even though you won't need extensive historical knowledge to design or renovate according to their principles, it will allow you to unearth the true purpose behind the different techniques mentioned throughout.

While the major focus of this book was on the principles of Vastu Shastra, Feng Shui is also relevant for many architects and people interested in learning more about the energy balance of their homes. You'll notice that you can combine many overlapping elements between the two sciences to produce something that is both convenient and original. Vastu has inspired a lot of Feng Shui's schools of thought, so drawing comparisons can show you the exact points of junction that you can take advantage of, especially about the concepts of Chi and Prana.

Most people who are interested in Vastu have turned to it because of their concern about the ecosystem. The modern world no longer has enough clean air and water for the environment to sustain itself and thrive. Vastu has become one of the go-to solutions for a growing number of modern designers and architects to reduce domestic and professional structures' carbon footprints. And while it'd be virtually impossible to force the whole world to utilize resources better, the more Vastu principles are applied, the more attracted people will become to its positive effects. The resources used today differ vastly from those that were used when these ancient sciences originated, but it shouldn't be too hard to find viable alternatives if you base your search on the principles of Vastu.

After learning about the pillars of Vastu, it's time to look inwards for ways to achieve the harmonious living you've just learned. No standard practice will miraculously make you feel in harmony, but you can always guide your steps with the balance acquired from Vastu and Feng Shui. You'll be able to associate the right elements with both your home and your workplace, and if you are an architect or an interior designer, you'll be able to effectively bring harmony and peace to the buildings and projects you'll be working on in the future.

Capturing the essence of Vastu can make you progress on a conscious level. Always use or follow those practices you understand, rather than comply with stale, outdated conventions. Relating its effects and causes will help you come closer to unlocking Vastu's true potential. Its principles can be applied virtually anywhere, whether it's a hut, factory, home, corporate offices, or even a school. It will be you who decides how to carry out them so it ensures a balanced energy dynamic.

Even though not all Sanskrit treatises have been translated to English because some were lost or produced in a dead language, there are plenty of resources that were unearthed and properly explain the major principles of Vastu. Many of the scriptures were considered at the time of writing this book to make sure that it's up-to-date with the latest translations. Also, it wouldn't be a bad idea to move on to researching specific treatises like the Manasara, Vastu Nirnaya, and many others after you've grasped the basics. If you've digested most or all the information in this book carefully, you may be ready to delve into more specific schools of thought on the ancient science of Vastu.

Since Vastu was created thousands of years ago, many interior designers and architects will find it challenging to integrate into their designs, but as you learn of the most popular methods and practices in use, you'll be able to intuitively do it because it's the natural order of things. Modern-day activities and quality of life are much more developed compared to their ancient counterparts, making it more of an interesting challenge to mix and match and strike that perfect balance using what you've learned in Vastu.

It might also be wise to integrate what you've learned about trees and green spaces whenever and wherever relevant. You should be able to understand why using Vastu Shastra to incorporate green spaces in your buildings is quite unique. There is no shortage of ideas you can implement in your home or workplace to help instill nature's vibrations in any space.

Novices may find it hard to keep up if they directly focus on implementing all the techniques and theories of Vastu Shastra. In this book, the slow-paced step-by-step guide format is enough to allow a beginner to catch up and get familiar with the concepts while still being straight to the point for users who've covered ground in this science before.

Avoid overwhelming yourself when you're trying to start Vastu Shastra in any location. It's important to understand that you must first be at peace with yourself before you can make your surroundings tranquil. Instead of recommending easier-said-than-done techniques, you won't encounter obstacles as you begin to explore the options at your disposal. From tearing down imprisoning walls to reorganizing a library, you should find the process meditative, liberating, and fulfilling.

Ultimately, as you implement the strategies detailed in this book, always remind yourself of your progress. Whether it was just a small renovation or a complete overhaul, you'll find it an enriching experience you just can't get enough of. Remember that taking well-defined and proactive steps will help you go through this life-changing experience, optimize your living spaces, and improve your physical and mental health.

Here's another book by Mari Silva that you might like

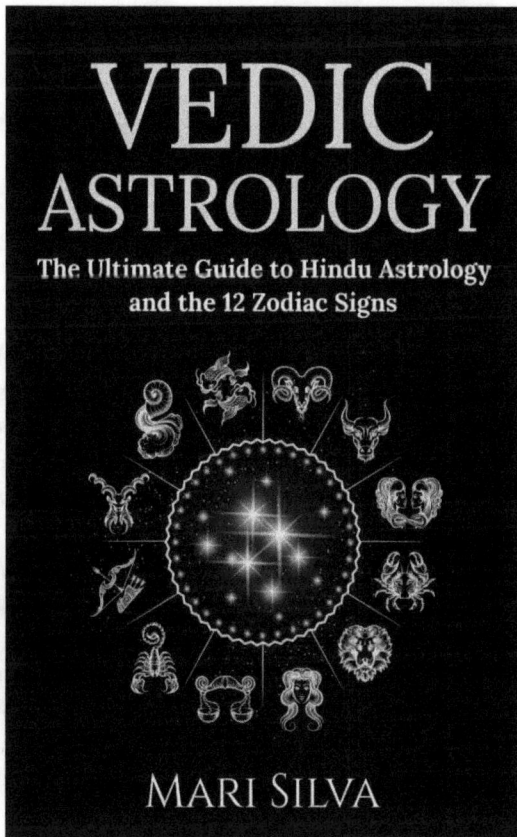

VEDIC ASTROLOGY

The Ultimate Guide to Hindu Astrology and the 12 Zodiac Signs

MARI SILVA

References

8 directions of vastu shastra and how they impact your life. (n.d.).
Www.Homeonline.com. https://www.homeonline.com/hol/home-tips/8-
directions-of-vastu-shastra-and-how-they-impact-your-life.html
10 Best Vastu Plants for Home. (n.d.). Www.Floweraura.com. Retrieved
from https://www.floweraura.com/blog/best-vastu-plants-for-home
20 Vastu tips to bring health and wealth in 2018 - Times of India. (n.d.).
The Times of India. Retrieved from
https://timesofindia.indiatimes.com/life-style/home-garden/20-vastu-tips-
to-bring-health-and-wealth-in-2018/articleshow/62118563.cms
*Benefits of Vastu Shastra | Importance of Vastu Shastra | Need for
Vastu Shastra.* (n.d.). Www.Prokerala.com. Retrieved from
https://www.prokerala.com/vastu-shastra/benefits-of-vastu-shastra.htm
Influence of Vastu on Modern Indian Architecture. (2020, August 4).
Center for Soft Power. https://www.softpowermag.com/influence-of-
vastu-on-modern-indian-architecture/
Karki, T. (2020, January 26). *Vastu tips: Sitting under pyramid roof
provides relief from insomnia, headache.* Www.Indiatvnews.com.
https://www.indiatvnews.com/lifestyle/vastu-vastu-tips-sitting-under-
pyramid-roof-provides-relief-from-insomnia-headache-583074
Livspace. (n.d.-a). *6 Simple Vastu Tips to Design Your Pooja Room.*
Livspace Magazine. Retrieved from
https://www.livspace.com/in/magazine/6-pooja-room-vastu-tips
Livspace. (n.d.-b). *6 Vastu-approved and Positive Colours for Your
Bedroom.* Livspace Magazine. Retrieved from
https://www.livspace.com/in/magazine/vastu-bedroom-color-as-per-vastu

Misconceptions about Vastu. (n.d.). Transcendence Design. Retrieved from https://transcendencedesign.com/blogs/vastu-blog/misconceptions-about-vastu

SCIENTIFIC VASTU PRINCIPLE | AAYADI (DIMENSION) | ARCHITECTURE IDEAS. (n.d.). Retrieved from https://architectureideas.info/2010/01/vastu-shastra-principle-aayadi-dimensions/

Vaastu Basics, Vastu Principles, Vaastu Shaastra, Vaastu India. (n.d.). Www.Vaastu-Shastra.com. Retrieved from https://www.vaastu-shastra.com/introduction-of-vastu-shastra.html

Vaastu Reference In Ancient Scriptures. (n.d.). Pandit.com. Retrieved from https://www.pandit.com/vaastu-reference-in-ancient-scriptures/

Vastu for office interiors: 10+ tips for success and prosperity at work. (2018, July 2). Architectural Digest India. https://www.architecturaldigest.in/content/vastu-shastra-office-success-financial-prosperity/

Vastu Purusha & Vastu Purusha Mandala [EXPLAINED]. (2014, March 6). Vastu Shastra Guru. https://www.vastushastraguru.com/vastu-purusha-mandala/

Vastu Purusha: The Fascinating Story. (n.d.). Www.Speakingtree.In. Retrieved from https://www.speakingtree.in/allslides/vastu-purusha-the-fascinating-story/brahma-asked-help-of-ashta-dikpalakas

VASTU SHASTRA. (n.d.). Www.Hinduscriptures.In. Retrieved from https://www.hinduscriptures.in/vedic-knowledge/vastu-shastra/vastu-shastra

Vastu Shastra: 10+ tips to attract good fortune with a garden at home. (2018, August 6). Architectural Digest India. https://www.architecturaldigest.in/content/vastu-shastra-garden-plants-good-fortune/

Vastu Tips: How To Attract Wealth To Your Home. (n.d.). Www.Makaan.com. Retrieved from https://www.makaan.com/iq/happy-home-family/vastu-tips-to-attract-wealth-to-your-home

What Is Feng Shui. (n.d.). The Feng Shui Society. https://www.fengshuisociety.org.uk/what-is-feng-shui/

What is Feng Shui? | An Interior Decorating Guide. (2017, September 11). Invaluable. https://www.invaluable.com/blog/what-is-feng-shui/

What is Vastu Pyramid and The Secret Behind It? (n.d.). Www.Magicbricks.com. Retrieved from https://www.magicbricks.com/blog/lifestyle/vastu/what-is-vastu-pyramid/115360.html

What is vital energy, or chi or prana? | Spiritual Therapies. (n.d.). Sharecare. Retrieved from https://www.sharecare.com/health/spiritual-therapies/what-vital-energy-chi-prana

What's the difference between prana and chi? (n.d.). Yogapedia.com. Retrieved from https://www.yogapedia.com/whats-the-difference-between-prana-and-chi/7/10313

12 most loved Yoga Sutras. (2018, April 4). YogaClassPlan.com. https://www.yogaclassplan.com/12-loved-yoga-sutras/

A Basic Introduction of Patanjali Yoga Sutras - Best Knowledge for Yogis. (2018, June 6). YogaMoha. https://yogamoha.com/introduction-of-patanjali-yoga-sutras/#i_Samadhi_Pada_51_Sutras

Ashtanga Yoga. (n.d.). Www.Yogapoint.com. Retrieved from https://www.yogapoint.com/ashtanga_yoga/yoga_sutra_1.htm

Ashtanga Yoga Classes in Mumbai | Shahzadpur Farm Yoga. (n.d.). Yoga Classes. Retrieved from https://www.shahzadpurfarmyoga.com/

Hewitt, I. (2015, June 13). *The Yoga Sutras 101.* The YogaLondon Blog. https://yogalondon.net/monkey/yoga-sutras-101/

Part 2, Introduction to Patanjali's Yoga: Samadhi-pada. (2013, July 3). Ekhart Yoga. https://www.ekhartyoga.com/articles/philosophy/part-2-introduction-to-patanjalis-yoga-samadhi-pada

Patanjali Yoga Sutras Explained with Meanings. (2019, October 9). Styles At Life. https://stylesatlife.com/articles/yoga-sutra/

Serving the Community of Lahiri Mahasaya Kriya Yoga. (2016, October 10). Lahiri Mahasaya Kriya Yoga. https://lahirimahasayakriyayoga.org/1-patanjali-yoga-sutra-samadhi-pada-or-samadhi-section/

Stern, A. (2019, February 26). *20 Particularly Relevant Yoga Sutras Translated and Explained.* YogiApproved™. https://www.yogiapproved.com/om/20-yoga-sutras-translated-and-explained/

The Chopra Center. (2018, August 24). The Chopra Center. https://chopra.com/articles/yoga-sutras-101-everything-you-need-to-know

The Most Important Yoga Texts | Yoga Guest Articles. (n.d.). Www.Sunnyray.org. Retrieved from https://www.sunnyray.org/The-most-autoritative-yoga-texts.htm

The Stages of Samadhi According to the Ashtanga Yoga Tradition. (n.d.). Yogainternational.com.

https://yogainternational.com/article/view/the-stages-of-samadhi-according-to-the-ashtanga-yoga-tradition

The Ten Most Important Sutras. (n.d.). Vito Politano. Retrieved from http://vitoyoga.com/tag/the-ten-most-important-sutras/

The Ten Most important Sutras - Judith Hanson Lasater. (2020, May 18). Feathered Pipe. https://featheredpipe.com/feathered-pipe-blog/yoga-sutras-judith-hanson-lasater/

The Yoga Sutras of Patanjali. (2019). Sacred-Texts.com. https://sacred-texts.com/hin/yogasutr.htm

What are the Yoga Sutras? (2018, November 28). BodyMindLife. https://www.bodymindlife.com/blog/yoga/what-are-the-yoga-sutras

Yanush Darecki. (2017). *Samadhi.* Yogananda.com.Au. http://yogananda.com.au/pyr/pyr_samadhi.html

Yoga. (n.d.). Yogapradipika. Retrieved from https://www.yogapradipika.com/

Yoga Meditation. (n.d.). Swamij.com. Retrieved from https://swamij.com/

Yoga Sutra. (2017, April 3). Yoga Journal. https://www.yogajournal.com/yoga-101/philosophy/yoga-sutras

Yoga Sutras. (n.d.). Swamij.com. Retrieved from http://swamij.com/yoga-sutras.htm

Yoga Sutras 101: Everything You Need to Know. (2019, August 24). Chopra. https://www.chopra.com/articles/yoga-sutras-101-everything-you-need-to-know

Yoga Sutras of Patanjali - Samadhi pada and Sadhana pada | Spirituality. (2018, March 31). Hindu Scriptures | Vedic Lifestyle, Scriptures, Vedas, Upanishads, Itihaas, Smrutis, Sanskrit. https://www.hinduscriptures.com/spirituality/yoga-sutras-of-patanjali-samadhi-pada-and-sadhana-pada/21016/

Yoga Sutras Of Patanjali Part 1. (n.d.). Thenazareneway.com. Retrieved from http://thenazareneway.com/yoga_sutras_of_patanjali_part_1.htm

www.ingramcontent.com/pod-product-compliance
Lightning Source LLC
Chambersburg PA
CBHW071956260326
41914CB00004B/816